# *Dangerous to Heal*

## Book One of The Displacement Duology

Also by Rebecca M. Zornow
*It's Over Or It's Eden*

# DANGEROUS TO HEAL

Rebecca M. Zornow

Dangerous to Heal

Text copyright © 2022 by Rebecca M. Zornow

This is a work of fiction. Names, characters, places, and incidents are either the product of the author's imagination or are used fictitiously. Any resemblance to actual persons living or dead, business establishments, events, or locales is entirely coincidental.

All rights reserved. No part of this publication may be reproduced or transmitted in any form or by any means, electronic or mechanical, including photocopy, recording, or any information storage and retrieval system without permission in writing from the author.

Requests for permission to make copies of any part of the work should be submitted online at www.RebeccaMZornow.com.

First Edition
978-1-7377118-5-8

*For Oliver,
who I want on
every adventure*

# Prologue

The journey home would start with one jump.

"We should get it over with," Hugo said, pushing impatiently at Elwen's side.

Elwen bristled and gave a dark look that Hugo didn't notice in the dim light. He shook off the dirty man and leaned over the long drop once more. Orange streaks of rust ran down the metal sides as far as Elwen could make out. Wind blew upward, giving life to the humid scent of decay and Elwen could guess what waited for them at the bottom should they fall. He straightened from his crouch and edged back.

Hugo nudged Michal and pointed to the length of pipes running alongside the tunnel on the other side of the chasm. "If we follow those, we'll eventually come to a maintenance area. We can swipe some uniforms—"

"And then what?" Michal croaked. He cleared his throat. "New clothes aren't going to get us off this crisping planet."

Hugo was steady against Michal's growing unease. "We'll see

what we find and make a plan. All I know is we can't stay here."

Michal shook his head a few times more than he needed to. "I can't jump that. You both are taller than me. There's no way I'll make it."

Elwen wanted to shake Michal and yell, *Well then, you should have stayed behind.* He was done with the fake solidarity. Done with waiting. He had to get out, now, no matter who got left behind. He wasn't going to waste his one chance because a blasted Hingarian had to stop and whine every step of the way.

Hugo looked back at the tunnel they emerged from, and his face crumpled in concern. And for good reason. "Listen," he spoke again to Michal, "it's far, but it's doable. I'll go first, so if you slip, I'll be there to pull you up."

The trio had already made it farther into the maze of service corridors and watershed passages than Elwen dared expect, but the victory of the immediate past paled in the face of what was coming next. It was time to act. Elwen was ready. He looked over the edge one last time and caught the scent of urine and shit on a powerful upward gust. His grimed sleeves blew against his arms, still well-muscled as his dubious trade called for. Akar Enterprises would mistreat and abuse but never in a way that would compromise the value of their assets.

That didn't stop their fourth cellmate from dying in the night. They woke to the gray tones of death and a medic came to remove the body. Elwen's own troubles left no room for the deceased, only those trying to survive—himself. Under the guise of helping the attendant wrap and prepare the body for removal, he lifted a digital key from the staff member.

It was a simple thing for a fine-fingered man who, until days ago, made his living as a professional thief on the tech planet of Onlo. In whispered tones, Elwen told Michal and Hugo what he had done but not from a place of generosity. He wasn't opposed to working with others if they better served his needs, unlike inflexible boneheads like, say, the first person who came to mind, his older brother who ran at first chance from the responsibilities of raising a kid sibling. Elwen was nothing if not practical. It was doubtful the others would sleep during his departure and—what was it they said? You didn't have to outrun the dösvengar, you just had to be faster than the slowest person.

Michal was still blubbering to Hugo. Elwen smiled. He had found his slowest person.

Hugo jerked back but not on account of Elwen's unspoken animosity. "Did you guys hear that?"

All three men snapped to attention. Was that the distant shuffle of running feet? Or water rushing?

"We need to go. Now." Hugo backed a few paces and stared intensely at the far side of the drop-off. He must have found something inside himself, for he jolted forward at a run and launched off his last footstep.

He was going to fall.

Hugo was going to hit the other side, a hand's width away from the surface—from freedom—and slide down, tumbling, tumbling down to whatever river of human waste lay out of sight.

Elwen shook his head as his mind caught up to the quick sequence of events. He had been sure Hugo was going to fall, but there Hugo was, on the other side, hoisting himself up, elbowing his way onto the dirty floor.

Hugo hadn't yet stood to his feet when Elwen was sure he heard something, some echo from the tunnels behind him.

Michal took no notice. "There's no way," he said. "You barely made it. There's no way I'm going to have a chance." In a perfect caricature, Michal sank to his knees, eyes locked on the escape route he'd never take.

Elwen looked down at the man and smiled. He'd jump, now that Hugo proved it possible. "Give the guards our regards."

"Give them yourself."

Elwen whipped around. His heart thundered yet there seemed to be a lack of blood in his brain. No, no, it wasn't possible. Elwen expected Akar guards to set on their trail like snarling, baying hounds, but how had they closed the gap so quietly?

The guard who spoke was flanked by two others in dark green, almost black uniforms. She smiled, much like Elwen had just smiled at Michal. He couldn't help but look behind, giving away Hugo's position, but the man was already gone.

"Don't worry," the guard said. "We'll catch your friend." Her viper hands were up and ready. In them were two tiny handguns.

Elwen cursed Michal in his head for delaying them all—and Hugo for selfishly leaving them behind—but was pleased to realize he wasn't afraid. He'd return to the cell. He'd find a new opportunity. He had instinctively crouched at the appearance of the guards—he was nearly as low as that bonehead Michal—and straightened in relief at the thought that there would be more chances. Akar could place him under higher security. They could even sell him. But he'd have the rest of his life to escape. Plenty of time for one as talented as him. Honestly, he almost felt calm at how things turned out. Hugo would likely slip and break a leg in these disgusting sewers, maybe even get shot as he tried to rush a cargo ship.

Elwen raised his hands in mock surrender as Michal blubbered at his feet.

The guard in charge led the way back through the tunnels, Elwen and Michal behind, the other two guards bringing up the rear. While running blindly, it felt like they were in the maze of tunnels for hours. In reality, it was a ten-minute walk to the edge of the service corridors. Long enough for Elwen to busy himself by watching the canvased ass of the guard in front of him.

The rounded, ever-shifting shape occupied only one side of Elwen's brain. The newfound realization that his escape was a matter of *when*, rather than *if*, was a welcome thought, but he still raged over the events that brought him to be captured and trafficked by Akar. He should have gutted Ranuel the moment she asked him to be fingersmith on the job she was pulling together. Or at least laughed in her face and gone for a drink instead. Had Ranuel been picked up as well? The thought brought a smile to Elwen's face. If only they crossed paths again in the Akarian underworld.

As the group rounded a corner, the confidence Elwen had so carefully crafted turned cold and melted down his spine.

Waiting for them were three gurneys.

"We didn't want to carry you." The guard raised her two guns once again. She didn't smile but cocked her head, as if Elwen was going to challenge her. As if he was going to fight her—an owned being herself, one utterly loyal to her master and fitting perfectly into her own small corner of the capitalist empire.

"You can't do this. I'm one of the best out there. Akar's bound to have clients that want the best thief money can buy." Why did Elwen's voice sound so far away? Why did she continue pointing the weapons at his chest? "You can't do this. Akar will lose on its investment."

She smiled, almost kindly. As if he were a small boy who did not understand the rules of the game he chose to play. Her voice purred, "You are a *very* minor asset. And now that you've proved yourself untrustworthy, you are worth more as parts."

Elwen took a breath to rebuttal as she pulled the trigger.

# Chapter 1

Yaniqui (*Yan-i-key*)
Agriculture Planet No. 4,278

Yaniqui lay in wait, hiding. The amber glow of sunset lit the normally dingy brown grasses until they shone like polished gold. Next to her, Sario's breath came faster than usual. Heat radiated off his sweaty body. She told herself not to look. To look at him would be the end of their friendship.

Instead, she watched the overseer's feet recede. She willed Fra Yu to walk faster even as she felt Sario's eyes on the mess of black curls that brushed her cheek. *Don't tuck it,* she willed Sario. *Don't you dare tuck my hair behind my ear.*

The older man's steps took him around the building's corner. Yaniqui risked a look at Sario, their waiting task thankfully pulling them out of the quiet, intimate moment. Her face broke into a smile of mischief and she tilted her head forward, goading him toward the office. Yaniqui pushed herself up and brushed debris from her faded waist wrap. Her back and thighs hurt from working all day in pale greenish-yellow dirt with a basket on her back, but it nearly didn't matter.

Yaniqui kept watch while Sario punched in the security code he had traded half his breakfast for. The door chimed and lifted Yaniqui's spirits.

They slipped into Fra Yu's office. Though routinely secured, there was little worth stealing inside the room. The chair and desk were made from thick ugly plastic. Dozens of overseers could use the same sturdy furniture and never need bother corporate with requests for new supplies. Yaniqui wasn't here for any of it. She was here for information.

The top drawer glided open beneath her fingers, and she pulled out a thin cylinder the length of her forearm. She slid the sides apart, one stick in either hand. When the right side unfurled fully, the empty air between each stick snapped to attention and became rigid. Words and images appeared, shimmering within the gap.

"Watch the door," she told Sario.

The holographic newsreel sputtered from poor connection and Yaniqui gave the sticks a soft shake. The fractured images stabilized into clear pictures. Yaniqui pretended to read the daily news, but when Sario turned his back, she performed a search: *H-L-O-B-A-N*. Then *B-A-Y-U-L, H-L-O-B-A-N*.

Her stomach gave a lurch when she saw a new search result, but it was only an article about a Shou University professor with a similar name. A few minutes more, and nothing satisfactory to be found. Yaniqui refitted the sides of the Loscroll together and replaced the cylinder in Fra Yu's desk drawer.

Sario turned at the sound of the drawer shutting. "And what in the news today was worth risking our meal vouchers for?" His smile belied his words. He'd give up twelve meals to wreak havoc with Yaniqui.

"Only a disappointing absence of information." Yaniqui shrugged a shoulder and spun on her boot toward the door.

Sario blocked her from leaving the dim room and at once the businesslike atmosphere of the break-in was replaced with a sort of sensual tension Yaniqui didn't care to have with her closest friend. He put a hand on his short brown beard in mock contemplation. "A disappointing absence of information?" he asked. "As in…the absence of an accepted application?"

Yaniqui took a sharp breath through her nose. The muted scent of plastic mingled with the ever-present scent of dust and telefungo paste. She frowned at Sario, ignoring his smile.

"How do you know about that?" She hadn't told anyone. Maemi wouldn't have either.

"A lot of people know you applied to university."

Yaniqui supposed that might be the case, but she wasn't sure how. "No, nothing's come through," she eventually said, sliding past him. "Maemi sent the letter a long time ago. I think it's as unlikely now as it was at the beginning."

She felt bad misleading Sario, but it was better he thought she was checking up on a university application than know who she was actually searching for. Like most things—including a single kiss, a too-harsh rebuff, one snappish mood from Maemi, or a wrestling match like the kind they had when she first arrived on 4,278—it would be the end of their friendship.

"Going to study would be a good opportunity," Sario said evenly, "but it's far away from everything you've ever known." He paused, chewing his hairless bottom lip, choosing words he hoped would matter. "There are advantages to staying here. Room to grow. I used to work in the fields, but now I'm part of the supply chain."

"This labor site isn't the only thing I know." Yaniqui's words dropped harsher than she intended.

She ducked her head out the door to glance down the dirt road. Empty. Everyone else was already heading to dinner.

Sario and Yaniqui fell silent as they walked the path to the common area. The brown-red soil of the planet's youth was all but gone. The ground was the color of sickness, a compilation of manufactured minerals, composted organic matter carted from the planet's largest moon, and pesticides. The crops Yaniqui cared for grew as well in the unnatural soil as they did in organic dirt. Better even. They were designed to.

The air still hung heavy between them when Sario murmured, "See ya," and peeled off.

It wasn't like him to let things go, so Yaniqui knew without a doubt her mother was approaching. Since arriving on the agricultural planet as indentured laborers, Maemi had never approved of "these wayward people you barely know who would betray you in an instant." Known to others as "friends."

"Yani, let us go," Maemi said, cutting off her daughter before she even started, "the food will run out." She was already glancing back to make sure Yaniqui was following. "I've been waiting to tell you all day," Maemi said when her daughter caught up. There was unfamiliar glee in her voice. "I saw a lizard today."

"Maemi, how can I believe that? Except for us, there's nothing bigger than a bug on this planet."

"And yet, it is true. The lizard was a brilliant green, not like these ugly leaves." Maemi gestured disdainfully at the crops. "She was missing a back leg and once she saw me, shot away as if the world was ending. Which, from her perspective, maybe it was."

Yaniqui felt herself taken in by the simple news. A moment ago, she didn't know the lizard existed but, as quick as discovery, optimism colored her mental image of a tiny lizard making a life for herself among the sea of crops.

"The fates will her safety," Yaniqui said.

"She's survived this long."

At the open-air canteen, a wide, low-roofed structure of corrugated tin and rare lumber shaded a few tables. The columns of the pavilion threatened anyone who dared lean on them with jagged splinters. There was no point in building anything more permanent as the laborers moved camp so often amid the plant ocean. The front tables were set with large pots of a pasty and filling mash, and small, manufactured packets of gel to make up the bulk of the workers' nutrition and caloric intake. One packet twice a day and one almost didn't need to eat. Almost—such an occurrence would have been a corporation's dream.

Once in line, Maemi straightened her own waist wrap, which was circled tightly around her pale yellow shirt. She pulled a stray thread off and rolled it between her fingers. "Yani, did you do your sums while working today?"

"Yes, Maemi. Square roots."

"What is the square root of 6,561?"

Yaniqui thought for some time as the line moved forward. "Eighty-one."

She was correct, but Maemi sighed. "We're so far behind. If only we had paper. Or more daylight." Maemi flung out her hand to the side, the way she did when she was frustrated. "What if our application comes through and we're not ready?"

Maemi always said *we* and *our*, but the scholarship was for Yaniqui.

In a discarded news scroll with paper so cheap it was nearly translucent, Maemi had read that two hundred and ninety less fortunate but promising indentured laborers were to be chosen to attend an adult education center on the twenty-third planet in the star system. The men and women selected would complete accelerated schooling to make up for years of education missed due to war, displacement, and general disruption.

Maemi had bleached the scroll in the sun so she could write over the top and saved her meager discretionary wages to post the letter, and her dreams with it.

It was remarkable that Maemi sent the application. Neither of the women had sent any voice recordings or other correspondence since Maemi first signed their labor contracts, Yaniqui having been underage at the time. They couldn't generally afford to send mail but that was secondary to the fact that there was no one to write to. Further, Maemi was fastidious about minimizing their exposure. But, as they closed in on a decade of working the grass seas of 4,278, Maemi became determined that her only child's story would not end there, rooting in the dirt. The only caveat was that, though Maemi didn't want Yaniqui to spend her life in a near Stone Age existence, neither did she want her daughter's identity exposed.

The line moved and Maemi prodded Yaniqui forward to take the bowl and packet Zimetta offered her.

From her own neatly tucked waist wrap, Yaniqui pulled out a curved piece of plastic to use as an eating utensil and sat on the ground with her mother. She often wished she could fling the wrap aside and let fresh air descend upon her navel, but the wraps were an essential part of their pretense. A proper Parentheite woman would never be seen in public without her waist wrap for fear that someone would see the desirable curve and round of her stomach. Parentheites thought it took two to spawn the sin of lust.

"What is a square root?"

"Maemi!"

"Okay, eat."

"A number that produces a specified quantity when multiplied by itself."

Maemi gave a part smile in response, but Yaniqui knew she did not grasp mathematics as well as her mother. She memorized what she was told but was inadequate all the while. Farming was tiring enough. There wasn't enough space in her head for the lessons Maemi wanted her to complete.

"It's important to be able to do mathematics mentally," Maemi said. She lowered her voice. "I saw a foreman last week who couldn't complete a sum in front of the overseer."

Yaniqui grinned sharply. "I'm guessing you were the only one scandalized in the situation."

They ate until an interruption came from the distribution tables. Yaniqui could barely make out, "There isn't any more," but Zimetta's gestures said more than enough. In front of her, the last of the line held dingy plastic cups, expecting water.

"Maemi, they're out of water." Yaniqui automatically licked her lips. They were dry. A painful crack opened in the middle of her bottom lip and immediately Yaniqui sucked on it.

"Hush, Yani," Maemi spoke softly.

Yaniqui felt the cut disappear. She looked around, but no one noticed.

Zimetta said, "That's all they gave us today. I cut the servings by more than half, but there's not enough."

"Why? What reason did they give for cutting the water rations?" Roh asked, his temper stoking itself in the hot, stale evening air.

Zimetta scowled back, unintimidated. There was a reason she was in charge of distribution at meals. "I would hope my job is worth more than that question."

Roh's powerful, knotted arms hung loosely at the sides of his sweat-marked shirt. He slammed the cup to the ground and walked heavily away on a stunted leg. The labor colony wouldn't feel the impact of a water shortage the next morning. They were feeling it now.

After dinner, Maemi and Yaniqui went to clean the dirt from their bodies as they normally did. That night, there was little water, and all of it dirty, barely fit for washing.

Yaniqui dipped her hand in the bucket of brown wash water. It wasn't enough for a full rinse but felt blessedly cool against her dry skin. She lifted her dark hair and wrapped her fingers around the curve of her sweaty neck. Limbs up and out, the fresh air felt good on the pits of Yaniqui's arms. The air smelled like bodies, but the simple odor of people wasn't unwelcome. On the heat-soaked world, the smell of humanoid sweat was ever present. It was the gritty dust stuck to Yaniqui's teeth that she wished gone.

Male voices carried over from the other side of the partition that satisfied a galaxy-wide law concerning laborers and their right to physical privacy. But it was really the grannies who stuffed grass in the gaps that protected the ladies' privacy. One mother crouched and washed the hands of a little boy and, though water rations were low, she splashed more water over the bug bites on his back, his tail swishing. Another child cried.

Yaniqui looked up. It was more than the whining of a child. Something was wrong.

Maemi stepped closer to the source and tugged on Yaniqui's faded sleeveless shirt to bring her along. Yaniqui pulled away but followed. She was curious who was hurt. It would be easier to not get involved, but she couldn't help the need to go and see what was happening.

Among the group of women—some Maemi's age and one so old her scalp peeked through her hair—Maemi and Yaniqui found a young girl with red eyes. Tears ran down her cheeks. Whereas Yaniqui's skin was a honeyed sand, the girl had the slightly silver look of the new recruits placed in Yaniqui's lodge only a few days ago. They came smelling fresh of loss, with few belongings and haggard eyes that barely saw their new work site. Whether they instead looked upon the packed inside of a slavecraft or the burning fields of their ancestors,

Yaniqui did not know. And she never would. Speaking of the raw past was near taboo. Best pretend it happened in a different life, or better yet, not at all. There was a limit for how much of another's pain you could absorb.

The last angled bit of sunlight set aglow a stripe of white down fur along the girl's shoulders and arms. It looked delicate against the tension of her small body, blistered and peeling hand cradled against her chest. Yaniqui felt a flash of empathetic pain when she guessed the problem. The girl touched the telefungo pesticide.

To keep the plants producing their starchy and long-lasting food, the workers had to apply a bright pink paste to deter the oblong beetles that burrowed into the inner edible part of the plant. It was a noxious concoction and dangerous to touch, but even more than indentured laborers who skipped out on their contracts or politicians in the Joint Council, the insects were the bane of agriculture corporations across the galaxy.

A woman with thick powerful legs and close-cropped hair dabbed at the girl's hand with a small cloth. The mother, Yaniqui assumed. Her eyes were purposefully neutral—this was just another hardship to bear, and less than the last—but her mouth was set.

"Here, here now. I've some salve. Made it from priscal egg and some good brown dirt," a short woman said, pushing her way through. Yaniqui vaguely recognized her. "My man was unloading the vats and one spilled down the side of his leg. We used this to heal the burn."

"Did it help?" The maemi spoke in a melodic whistle.

Belatedly, Yaniqui realized it wasn't a song, but an unusual accent.

The short woman had no trouble understanding but paused, as if searching her recollection. She scratched at the bites along her wrist, the result of angry beetles. "Well, not so. But his was quite more severe, see. Your girl has a little burn. Maybe the salve will work faster for her." The squat woman carefully scooped paste from an old tin container and handed it to the mother. "I'm off to see him now. He's in the infirmary."

The mother smelled the wet mixture before applying it lightly to her daughter's hand.

Maemi caught Yaniqui's eye and nodded toward the lodge. It was on putrid yellow soil like everything else, but the women took turns sweeping morning and night, slowly packing the dirt hard and shiny. Yaniqui had slept there before, not only the few nights previously, but on and off during the past nine planting seasons. It was the same routine each time they moved in—pound the walls to scare out arachnids, stomp them, sweep the floor, and lay out the mats. A few days later, they moved to another set of fields.

The light was nearly gone and most of the other women, girls, and small boys were inside. Maemi and Yaniqui pulled off their clothes. Yaniqui learned long ago not to be self-conscious in a roomful of women. When the waist wrap came off and the stuffy air of the lodge hit her freed stomach, it transformed into a delicious fresh breeze. The sin of lust be damned. It felt good to bare her navel.

The wrinkled stretch marks on Maemi's stomach pulled taut as she slid her sleeping smock overhead. Yaniqui did the same and went outside to beat their tunics, trousers, and waist wraps. She was so hot she didn't care who saw her in her smock without her wrap on. It was nearly dark besides. A faint halo of dust appeared, and she coughed.

Yaniqui folded the clothes and put them at the foot of the mat she slept on with Maemi. At every new shelter, Maemi pushed to be first in and placed their mat in the corner. It had the most privacy and was farthest from the door. No one going out to relieve themselves at night would step over them.

She stretched out on the ground and closed her eyes. The precious few moments before sleep were the only ones Yaniqui had to herself. She spent them drawing forth memories of the life and home she had long ago, embellishing what she had forgotten or never had the opportunity to experience.

There was a familiar whimper. Yaniqui opened her eyes. The little girl with the chemically burned hand lay curled on the other side of the dim shack. Zimetta's eldest daughter was trying to calm the mother. Yaniqui could hardly understand what the mother said in response, but the statements from Zimetta's daughter made it clear that not only did the girl's hand get burned, but her gloves were also ruined. And the mother was just learning that those ripped gloves would be tracked back to the family to become another debt.

Maemi, who wasn't yet lying down, went over and put a finger on the mother's wrist, topaz against silver. "Friend, it is hard to be here. Hard for us all. We know this."

Yaniqui's jaw tensed. Her mother always did this when someone was in trouble. The neutral statement. The threadbare acknowledgement of pain felt. Weak gestures.

Maemi tried to explain it to Yaniqui once—it was more than that. It was an acceptance of hardship that could not be changed. A gesture of empathy. But Yaniqui knew they could do more.

When Maemi came back to lie down, Yaniqui whispered, "That little girl, we could—"

"No. If you help her, someone wonders how. That is the end."

Yaniqui rolled over to face the wall.

"I know," her mother said, more gently. "It is hard when another suffers something that we could take away. Even then, that still would not mean that *you* don't suffer in their place. And, in this new existence, it means you will eventually suffer many times over."

There was often someone in the labor colony sick or hurt. Adults took it in stride. They knew suffering lingered in the rotten food, a brace of knuckles, or even the sun above them. It was the little ones who were the hardest to watch in those moments. They cried and hung on to their maemis or their mamas or their mems. The despair and confusion clear in their wails: Why is this happening to *me*?

It bothered Yaniqui so much because she could help, more than anyone expected.

"Maemi…"

"No, go to sleep. I will know if you get up."

Yaniqui closed her eyes, shutting out her mother and the simple dormitory around her.

Her thoughts alighted on the image of a man.

The sun scorched by midday. Yaniqui wore gloves covered in pink telefungo paste, so she couldn't even slip a finger under her waist wrap to air it out. Using her shirt to shade her head like many of the men were doing was a faraway dream. The crops were tall but thin, and they provided only the barest of shade patches. A thin drip of sweat ran down her temple when a woman's shout came from a few rows over.

Yaniqui peered through the stalks in Maemi's direction, but she was so far ahead, she couldn't see her. Yaniqui carefully rolled off her gloves. She jogged down the row, taking care around the freshly pinkened plants.

She left the shelter of plants and entered a clearing. An older man lay on the ground like a crumpled cloth. Next to him was a pile of infested stalks set to burn. Intuition told Yaniqui the elder was tired and thirsty, not sick or hurt. Water would perk him up like a wilted plant, if they could find it. She nodded at two others that had just arrived that she would help carry him out of the brush. He was a small man but his limp condition made it slow going. He moaned when the group stopped to adjust their hold. They flagged the nearest foreman, Roh, and the group made for an electric vehicle. Roh's curbed gait kept him in time with them as they carried the man.

Roh gestured at Yaniqui. "Get in, Yaniqui. Make sure he doesn't slide out." The transporter was the most basic of vehicles with little more than wheels, an engine, and a flat space for hauling supplies or people. Despite the man's immediate situation, Yaniqui was thrilled to leave the fields behind. Within seconds, a tantalizing breeze circled her. Yaniqui held on to the man with one hand while the other pulled her hair back to let the sweat dry. Yaniqui was surprised to see the man wasn't sweaty. She touched his neck. Clammy. It was definitely heatstop. He was still breathing but shallowly. Yaniqui loosened the man's shirt and tried to shade his face from the sun, but what he needed was water. Yaniqui glanced sharply at Roh to make sure he wasn't looking back, and then moved both her hands to the man's chest. She could help him make it through, but he still desperately needed to drink.

They drove along the massive farms, all with the same burly stalks. Identical fields lined the planet for as far as Yaniqui could see. She knew there were mountains somewhere on the world, but no one had yet come up with a way to effectively farm them. The only thing she liked about the planet was the huge moon visible by day. A long green mountain range ran down one side. Word was they were mining that though. Eventually it would be gone.

Roh drove toward a small collection of permanent stone and metal buildings. Yaniqui didn't have much reason to visit them, but they weren't unfamiliar. They were flat and stark because the corporation refused to spend on frivolous design. At the single-story infirmary, Yaniqui and Roh picked up the man, brought him in, and laid him down on a cot. Roh pulled off the man's shoes and nodded his thanks at Yaniqui. A young woman Yaniqui had never seen before came and set to work on the rest of his clothing.

Yaniqui looked away. The beds—real cushioned beds—were dotted with patients.

She started when she saw Sario sitting on one of the beds. His shirt was off. He waved her over and she took in the bloody gash on his arm. There was no doubt, even injured, there was a strong elegance in those arms.

"It's fine," he reassured her. "Jamison lost grip of a crate he was passing down to me."

Yaniqui stared a bit too long at his bare shoulders and Sario smiled, his eyes never leaving her face.

"I should get back," Yaniqui said, clearing her throat. "See you tonight."

"Always."

Yaniqui pretended she hadn't heard that last bit as she walked to the door. No longer distracted by hauling the older man in, she caught sight of the little girl with the name of a whistle. Yaniqui wasn't surprised. The kid whimpered throughout the previous night. In the bright morning, the mother gave a shocked cry when she saw how red and tender the hand had grown in the span of one sleep cycle.

Yaniqui glanced around, but everyone in the infirmary was occupied.

"Hi," Yaniqui whispered tentatively. She moved closer. "I know you're new, but we stay in the same lodge. How's your hand?"

The girl looked down and didn't seem like she was going to answer. Suddenly, tears slipped out and the girl's chin quivered. "It's so hot. But I—they said it's infected." The words had an unusual quality to them, but she was easier to understand than her mother. "They said I might lose my hand." More tears spilled.

Yaniqui's heart fell for the girl. Life without a hand in an indentured labor colony would be terrible. The girl would never be able to produce, never pay off her contract. As a child, every opportunity was supposed to be in front of her, not gone before it began.

*Hloban, I'm going to do it.*

"Can I see it?" Yaniqui asked.

"Don't touch it!" the girl panicked. "It hurts so bad." She sniffed back a bubble of snot.

"I'll be careful."

Grudgingly, the tiny girl nodded and Yaniqui took her silvery hand in hers. The stripe of white down fur ended at her wrist. Yaniqui lifted the bandage slightly and peeked under. Inflamed crimson skin stretched across her palm.

"Do you know what planet your people come from?" Yaniqui asked.

The little girl looked up and Yaniqui continued to hold her hand.

"Vertue." She stopped crying.

"Have you ever been there?"

The child shook her head. "I was born on a cargo shuttle. My mimmi says Vertue has delicious birds to eat and grass with plump heads you can suck on."

Yaniqui let her fingertips slide beneath the bandage and concentrated. She felt the dying, charred cells in the skin and muscle. The swarm of infection. In the hollow of Yaniqui's collarbones, she felt an echo of the girl's pulse and the pain that raced through her body. Yaniqui's hands warmed and she felt the pull of agony as the pain became fully realized in her own body. Faint at first, but then it grew. Yaniqui fought to keep her expression blank. Black curls fell into her face, but she didn't stop to push them aside.

The girl sniffed and looked sharply at Yaniqui under hooded eyes. Yaniqui let go and wiped a sleeve down the side of her own sweaty face. The girl pulled her bandage down and inspected her wound. The red was now pink, the open sore was half the size, and the pus of infection dissipated.

Yaniqui did not want to push it too far. It was better if it seemed like a natural turnaround.

"It's a secret, okay?" Yaniqui whispered.

The little girl nodded in a tired way; her energy was sapped by the fast transformation.

"I hope you feel better." Yaniqui patted the girl's outstretched calf as her small friend settled into a nap. Warmth lingered in Yaniqui's hands. She already knew she would not tell Maemi what she had done.

Even in the sun for three seconds, Yaniqui missed the shade of the building. It would be tiresome to walk back on foot. She glanced around and walked to either side of the infirmary, but Roh was nowhere in sight. She would have to catch up on her work and be late to dinner. Maemi would help her after her own quota was reached, but she would glare. Maemi didn't approve of anything that brought notice upon them.

Yaniqui started on the road back and a hand snaked out of the tall crops to touch her elbow. She looked in surprise at Sario's face, grinned, and followed him in. It took a few steps more to realize Sario wasn't playing. Neither did he have the air of intensity he got before trying to kiss Yaniqui.

He was mad.

"Why didn't you tell me?"

Yaniqui cocked her head. "About the university application? It's not real. It's never going to happen."

Sario closed the gap between them. His breath came hot on her cheek as he struggled to keep his voice down.

"I saw you in there with that girl. And I've seen you before." Sario frowned.

Yaniqui frowned too. She knew Sario was always watching. Perhaps she hadn't understood how closely.

"You come up to a kid, and their tummy feels better a few moments later. Or someone's fever goes down. That...that girl's hand. I checked it after you left. It did not look like that minutes ago when the nurse changed her bandage. The kid was howling so loud the plants shriveled, but now she's just...what? Fine?" He swallowed. When

Yaniqui didn't say anything, he asked, "Why didn't you tell me what you could do?"

Yaniqui took a deep breath. How could she ever have told Sario?

Yaniqui *was* gifted. But her planet was gone—and there was nothing in the universe to protect her. Sario knew that. Everyone on the labor planet was intimately acquainted with the desperation and vulnerability displacement brought.

What Sario didn't know was there were mega-trillionaires in Selruit that would hire Yaniqui for her services. Medical labs would skin her to the bone seeking the source of her people's power. Corporations like Akar Enterprises would compete to enslave her, not as an indentured laborer on a farm, but as a true slave in all but name.

Sario rubbed a hand back and forth across his beard in frustration. "Yani, there's no denying it. I *know*. Roh probably does too. He's always asking for you to help move people when they're sick."

She turned away from Sario and stared at the thicket of leaves to her right. She took a breath and thought quickly. Discovery was Maemi's nightmare, not hers. Sario was her oldest friend. He was already part of her story. And, more than anything, Yaniqui believed in fate. She had a good story coming to her.

"Yes, it's true," Yaniqui said shakily in spite of her decision to be honest. "I can heal people because I'm Wea Saavian. But you can't tell anyone."

The resentment lifted from Sario's eyes. "Of course not."

Yaniqui reached out and lifted his bandage. Sario's lips parted in surprise when she put her hand on the gash. It warmed and she felt the raw, bloodied edge of cut flesh. The prick of each dissolvable stitch. It wasn't a bad injury and it didn't take long to heal.

Sario inspected it in disbelief and Yaniqui smiled. It was nice being able to heal someone fully and see their honest response. "Oh crisps, Maemi can't know you know either."

A husky chuckle escaped Sario as the elation of a shared secret caught up to him. "As if Nica knew half of what we get up to."

"I mean it. This might seem fun to you. But it's not." She read the question in his eyes. She whispered, "There is no protection for a person like me."

He very nearly rolled his eyes. "It's like that for everyone here. That's *why* we're here."

How could she tell him about the risks she faced as a woman without the protection of a home? How could she tell him about the burden of being able to heal but being too scared to use it? About Wea Saavian fate?

"I'm not being a princess about it, Sario. I can heal my own body; I can heal—truly heal—another person's body. I've got...I've got this gift to do good, but the ironic thing is I can't help people. Not really." She put her hand on top of her head in thought and to shield her part from the blistering sun. "If I used my abilities freely, I'd be discovered and taken. Used."

Sario looked away from the intensity in Yaniqui's eyes, but she pushed his shoulder back and made him listen to what Maemi had drilled into her head over the past ten years.

"The thing about nice things is everyone wants them for themselves."

# Chapter 2
Ippa *(E-pa)*
Shou University

<u>Galactic Anthropology Final Paper, Level One</u>
Earth, a small habitable planet in the Sol System, has been facing systemic extinction of its species and cultural richness since it made Contact with the larger galaxy.

The planet is 4.6 billion Earth years old. Its surface is 75 percent water and its atmosphere is 78 percent nitrogen, 21 percent oxygen, 0.093 percent argon, and 0.04 percent carbon dioxide. Humanoids, animal creatures, and flora inhabit the surface and oceans but there are no Intelligent animoid species on-planet. After Discovery, or more likely a level six Rediscovery, there was initial speculation about dragons, but it is clear the now-extinct Earth reptiles were non-Intelligent, similar only in size to dragons.

From historical tales in the oral tradition, backed by DNA analysis, it is hypothesized that a moderately sized spacecraft from another star system landed on Earth as part of the Black Wars Migration. These travelers either purposefully decided to inhabit the planet or could not relaunch after exploring. In either case, the travelers found the remote planet habitable and a refuge from the War. It would be two hundred thousand Earth years before their descendants made off-planet Contact again.

The humanoid explorers' arrival triggered the demise of the only Intelligent life on-planet: humanoid-like Neanderthals and closely related species. The Neanderthals were wiped out due to competition for resources, or else forcibly killed off, but not before the two groups intermixed. Some present-day Earth populations have approximately 2 percent Neanderthal DNA. This extinction is an epitome of the risks of colonizing planets before localized species reach their full potential.

Over generations, both knowledge of life off-planet and advanced technology were largely lost. Though the travelers came with advanced thought and skill, their descendants lived in a technology-barren world. As the general population grew, they were forced to follow the traditional path from Stone Age to Iron and Bronze, and, finally, to Space Age.

Four generations ago, when Earth sent a manned spacecraft to the end of the Sol System, it was met by a First Contact Delegation from the Joint Council, per the regulations of Protective Decree 894.7. One ambassador noted in his report, "When we boarded the Earthlings' spacecraft, one of their party bowed down in reverence, five led an attack against us, and the last regurgitated fluids and food particles."

After Contact, Earth began to trade, primarily in salt water and plant seeds. The Joint Council added two Earth delegates for input and knowledge transfer but did not grant voting privileges. It is fair to say that Earth is a spectator of, not a participant in, modern-day events.

With this new tie to other civilizations, Earth quickly enhanced its technology, however anecdotes demonstrate the population struggles to maintain their historical traditions. Youth in particular readily adopted foreign tastes in music, clothing, and language. Bound paper books gave way to popular holographic drama; bicycles, an important form of transportation, became near obsolete.

Now that every Earthling alive has never known a time before Contact, it is difficult to—

**Ippa leaned back in her chair and stretched her arms behind her head, working the kinks out of her shoulders as she proofread her paper on the obscure planet, hopefully for the last time. She hit something**

solid and warm. Ippa sat up and turned in her chair, maybe slower than she would have if she had gotten a full night's sleep.

"Sorry about that," Ippa said.

Another Level One looked back at her with tired eyes, hardly registering her apology. He turned back to his work: three thick volumes filled with tiny print, one open to a diagram. Whether it depicted the internal organs of some creature's body or a map, Ippa could not tell.

Ippa turned back to her own dense books and ran a fingernail along the piping of her university-issued jacket. She knew she should stop—the white piping was taking on a gray tinge from being handled so much. Her final project, which included a paper, presentation, and annotated bibliography, was a huge undertaking. If it wasn't for the resulting evaluation, it would be a relief to turn the paper in to be done with it.

A tight feeling rose in Ippa's chest as she realized the chairs around her were filled. How long had she been sitting there double-checking the compositions of a planet's atmosphere she would never visit? She strained her bleary eyes at the horizontal timepiece on the wall. Quicksilver poured back and forth between chambers as fluid as the march of time.

What the timepiece read—that she was late—was the only thing that could have electrified Ippa in her fatigued state. She scooped everything off the work surface and into her bag, only taking care with her university holo. The chair collapsed smoothly and effortlessly under the table.

Space was at a premium in the biblioplaza. It was as if hundreds of pack rats spent millennia saving books and scrolls and electric type and every other thing that could be scrounged up from across the galaxy. Academic pack rats. Workspaces were an affront to a slice of floor that could otherwise be used to catalog Zarbon period dramas.

Ippa bumped into the young man behind her again.

"Sorry, sorry. So tight in here. You know, all the books," Ippa said, barely glancing at the other student.

She zipped toward the exit as fast as possible but an excess of information made it difficult to navigate. The worktables were packed tightly, but she didn't want to venture into the maze of shelves and drawers. So far, her first year as a student seemed equally focused on memorizing the layout of the university as it did on learning.

Shou University or "The Shou" as many in the know called it (and Ippa was delighted to count herself among them), was a huge metropolis of study and research, the biggest and most prestigious in the galaxy. The acceptance rates were so miniscule they were almost nonexistent. Ippa reminded herself several times a day it was a privilege to study there. The Shou specialized in "the intricacies and absoluteness of the connective resource." Or the study of the galaxy. It was the only university that looked at the galaxy from a comprehensive perspective. Ippa did not want to learn how to engineer spaceships or how to manage agricultural workers. She wanted to know everything.

At the front of the great hall, a wave of warm dry air came through when someone exited the front doors. Never hot, never cold, the planet had the ideal weather for preservation of texts and samples. The university had acquired the planet before there were beings on Earth.

Ippa glanced at the timepiece again. There was no way around it. She was going to be late.

*Zzzzzzzzzzzzzzzzzzzzzzzzzzzzzzzzzzzzzzzzzzzzzzzzzzzzzzzzzzzzzz zzzzzzzzzzzzzzzzzzzzzzzzzzzzz* "Oh crisping papers," Ippa said, but no one could hear her over the buzz. *Zzzzzzzzzzz*

*Zzzzzzz* The AI guard clonked over on thick robotic legs and shouted in competition with the alarm, "Did you visit the registrar?" though the answer was obvious. *Zzzzzzzzzzzzz*

*Zzzzzzzzzzzzzzzzz* "I-I'll go now." *Zzzzzzzzzzz*

The guard swiped his hand over a sensor to quiet the alarm and moved forcefully in front of the exit, as if Ippa was going to bolt, still in unlawful possession of the heavy books. The guard was an old AI model with a stern but not quite humanoid expression on its face. Ippa had a wild and absurd impulse to laugh.

"Leaving without registering books is a serious offence," the guard recited. "The Shou biblioplaza has over 14,002,300,000 manuscripts, books, holos, scrolls, carvings, and texts. If you remove one of the resources without proper registration, you are subject to a five hundred yurr fine and required to appear before the Disciplinary Committee."

Ippa backed away from the entrance. The guard's heavy brows dipped together, black lines making a point. Ippa covered her mouth to keep from laughing and said as seriously as she could, "I know. It was a mistake."

She turned on the heel of her boot, only to find every head in the hall looking at her. She had three hundred eyes on her easily. Plus a few extra from the large animoid in the corner. The urge to laugh dried up.

Ippa could not believe she forgot such a standard requirement as registering a book. She knew the rules, obviously. Everyone had attended the exhausting training session on utilizing the biblioplaza at the start of the year.

Ippa expected life at The Shou to be demanding, but she never imagined this. Between class sessions and work activities, there was hardly time to complete assignments. Her mind was growing more and more like the biblioplaza itself. There was hardly room left for Ippa.

She marched up to the desk, acutely aware of being watched. She put her bag on the counter and pulled out one, two, three, four, five, six books.

The attendant sniffed and asked, "Six books?" as if she hadn't witnessed the scene at the doors.

"Yes, I know. Six books on an obsolete planet I'll never see."

The attendant settled into a bland yet severe stare. "Shall I return them to the cabinets for you?"

"Uh, no, please register them to my account." Ippa blushed, making her heavy collection of freckles stand out, and she stacked the books in her bag for the second time. She avoided looking anywhere but the door—it was better not to know if hundreds of her peers were still watching her.

Ippa hurried along the perimeter of the biblioplaza. She did not run. Running was undignified, a clear indicator of poor time management, and Ippa would never allow herself to be labeled guilty of such, but she did keep a brisk pace, eyes locked on Burteno Hall as if she could will it closer. She jogged up the steps of the building as casually as she could.

She found Room B21 and entered to find the other students already fulfilling their out-of-class responsibilities. They sat at tables wearing digital analysis glasses as they cataloged recently acquired specimens and samples.

Ippa glanced at the containers resting on carts along the wall. Some samples were already marked. Her lateness was disrespectful to the other students and she had missed any important information the facilitator had given at the beginning of the session. This was happening too regularly lately. Things would have to change.

Ippa took a place at the table and slipped on a pair of glasses. A simple navigation menu came up on the lens. Ippa slowly and carefully removed a slide from a small box. She selected the magnifier on her glasses with a flick of her iris and adjusted the focus with a movement of her hand.

"Ippa," Bel, the girl next to her, whispered. "Did you get the message from Professor Jinu?"

Ippa did not look up but said, "About the paper format?" She wrote a description on an adhesive label.

"No, about the live sources. Jinu wants us to interview a source from our planetary assignments." Bel took off her glasses and licked an eyeball with her tongue. Almost as an afterthought, she licked her large, rounded glasses too.

Bel was part of the 3 percent of the student body made up of animoid beings. The university was notorious for keeping them out. Many cried speciesism, but the university stated that it was simply a matter of logistics. They did not have the time (or the inclination) to widen doorways or install tanks for water-based creatures or grow blooms of gold algae for species that ate only such. As it was, Bel was not allowed near the paper texts—no amphibians were. The saving grace in her application for study was her ability to discern ultraviolet rays.

Ippa looked up sharply. "But it's just supposed to be an annotated write-up of previously collected information," she said. Ippa didn't want to admit the whine that crept into her voice.

"I know, I know." Bel set her slide down and made a subtle double click in her throat. "Ippa, there's only twelve people on the planet I was assigned. What if someone died since the census was taken and the population was cut by 8.33 percent? What if there was an epidemic? I won't have anyone to interview."

Ippa had never seen Bel unsettled before. Amphibians have notorious poker faces, but there was a gray tinge to the yellow spots on her cheeks.

"It's due tomorrow. Why is Jinu adding something now?" Ippa asked. She was hit by a self-generating mental list of the extra steps she would have to take after the work session instead of sleeping. The slide tumbled out of Ippa's hands and fell to the floor. The quiet sound of shattering glass rang through the room. Bel gasped. Everyone turned to look at Ippa, astonished at her blatant disrespect of university material.

"And that's why planet Ina of the Induea System has the most diverse array of life in sixteen major forms."

"Thank you, Lemworth. High praises. Next is Ippa, speaking on a little planet called Earth," Professor Jinu said. Jinu nodded at Ippa and made a quick calculation on her view-protected holo, recording Lemworth's score. Jinu's long face showed no hesitancy. She was faster than any computer when it came to deciding the academic value of her students.

Professor Jinu said she assigned inhabited planets randomly to the Level One class of a thousand students, but Ippa was sure she picked favorite students to pair with the most interesting planets. And in her subsection class of a hundred, Ippa was the one assigned Earth.

Ippa walked to the front of the room, tired from her late night. She managed to make contact with a woman on Earth named Loera who was willing to be interviewed. Loera's husband was originally from off-planet so she had an interesting perspective. Her answers were clear and concise and it was easily one of the most fascinating things that had happened since Ippa started Level One at The Shou, but she was nearly too exhausted to listen. She only hoped the interview quotes she added to her paper in her fatigue-addled state made sense.

Ippa's hand shook slightly as she started her presentation. All she had to do was perform the required gestures in front of the sensors to access her personal folder. Ippa wanted a holographic image of Earth to appear, showcasing the large blue oceans and white cloud patterns. She gestured and instructor feedback from Molecular Understanding appeared instead. *Your analysis of the second study sample is lacking.* A murmur ran through the learning hall.

"Sorry," Ippa gasped. She did the proper hand motion to start her presentation.

Ippa checked that the proper image was displayed and began, "Earth is the third planet in the Sol System, located in the Orion Spiral Arm."

Ippa watched her holographic representation of Earth, written in her own code, spin slowly. Her short blue hair was sure to look brilliant next to the large oceans. Ippa spotted a tiny land bridge between two continents she was particularly fond of. It was a miniscule curve, but that little piece of land provided animals with additional territory to explore and challenged humans when they began traveling by seacraft. At a Thought Prioritization Examination, her advisor told her this type of distractive thought would never benefit her academic career. She had to focus.

"Ippa? We're waiting for the presentation." Professor Jinu frowned.

The ghost of Earth floated in the dim room and ninety-nine students stared at Ippa, who realized belatedly she had stopped speaking.

Ippa took a deep breath and stumbled through an explanation of the physical characteristics, the story of life, and the current culture and technology on Earth. She fingered the piping on her jacket as she looked at her peers. It was hard to make out their faces in the darkened room. She caught a glimmer of light on someone's glasses, but no one nodded along or smiled at Ippa. Oh crisps—was her jacket fraying?

"I still don't know what Earth is. I know the makeup of its soil and the basic DNA structure for life on the planet, and what cacti are, but I don't know what the planet *is*." Ippa realized too late she said something best left in the back of her mind. The class, already quiet, went still at the admission of ignorance.

The professor cleared her throat but stayed seated. Ippa saw a momentary reflection off Jinu's smart contacts, technology banned from the student population. "Ippa, your statement does not add up. You had the allotted time in your schedule to research Earth and examine the samples we have. I believe there were three?" Professor Jinu said.

"Four. Jellyfish, cockroach, and mouse, all animals representing a different aspect of organic life on the planet, but I included Earthlings as they share a common ancestor with one of the Original Nine of Intelligent life."

Jinu leaned forward. "But I know for a fact we don't have an Earth human sample."

"No, but we have samples of humanoids from the Original Nine. I wrote a program to analyze how the DNA might have changed based on Earth's environment."

"You did original theoretical analysis of Earth?"

"Yes, Professor Jinu." Ippa tried to keep the pride out of her voice.

"That wasn't part of the assignment," Jinu said, not unkindly, "but regardless, wouldn't it follow that you did the project, Ippa? Why did you say you 'do not know the planet?' We heard your summary. You contacted the live source. Did you not do a thorough job?"

"I did. I know that the Earth humans created over five hundred species of something they call a dog through selective evolution. By picking the animals that were kindest and smartest, they created a collaborative relationship with a species of their own design."

"Ippa—"

Ippa knew this was going wrong, but her head was so foggy she felt insulated against the logic telling her to stop.

"—I know that the planet has so many varied ecosystems, there's a reptile called a chameleon and one subspecies lives only on one small, rocky islet and nowhere else." Ippa knew she was speaking too fast and willed herself to slow down, but she couldn't. "I know that no one yet knows how many beetles exist on Earth, but there's a tiny creature called an ant that looks *exactly* like a quimbar from Planet 24 and no one knows why. The more we know, the less we know *why*.

"Are all of these occurrences the result of random pieces of cosmic dust that drifted together to create something extraordinary but meaningless?" Ippa was relieved to get this out and connect with her classmates on a different level. They spent so much time rushing; they rarely talked about why they did the work they did and what they hoped to do with it.

"*Ippa.*" Professor Jinu finally broke through Ippa's monologue. "None of that was the assignment. The assignment was to create a paper, presentation, and annotated bibliography of information the university has on Earth, and add one new interview to the lineup."

"Which I did, but I was curious about what we don't know," Ippa said. The Earth spun lazily in the darkened room even as a wave of anxiety came over Ippa.

"Ippa, go to my study and wait there. We have lost valuable time in this conversation. Time from each of the one hundred people here. And I suspect I will lose more of my time to you before this day is over."

The class tittered quietly enough that Ippa couldn't identify a single person who laughed. Ippa made out Bel in the second row, stoic as always. Another student was already approaching the front for their presentation. There was nothing to do but collect her bag. Her face grew warm and she left the classroom. She never heard of a student being sent from a session before.

Professor Jinu's office was in the oldest wing of one of the oldest buildings on campus. It was dry and sterile, and every time Ippa entered, her ears pressurized when the door closed behind her. She walked down the hall and opened the door to Professor Jinu's study. On one wall was a shining beacon of star systems, seemingly floating, reaching beyond where Ippa knew the wall had to be. The depth and detail were beautiful. Ippa walked up to it and hesitated before reaching out a hand and spinning the model until her home star system appeared.

Ippa thought of her family's investment in her dream and the sacrifice it had taken to get this far: memorizations and scholarship requests and forgoing her fourteenth birthday ceremony so she could attend a lecture from a visiting professor. Mother was so upset with her that day. *If you spend your entire life studying life, you are going to miss your own.*

Ippa's eyes had burned since she woke up that morning and her ears throbbed uncomfortably. Her body was heavy and dumb. Suddenly, Ippa felt like she had never had a break before in her academic-fueled life. She sank into one of Professor Jinu's sling chairs, rested her head on the back, and closed her eyes.

*Thwack.* Professor Jinu slammed her palm against the intricate depiction of the galaxy on the wall. Ippa bolted upright and stars, planets, and comets disappeared with a strange sucking sound underneath Jinu's hand. Jinu's face was usually composed, but her green eyes blazed and her lips were set in a thin grimace. The calm of the classroom was gone.

It came rushing back to Ippa. The failed presentation. The public admonishment.

Some pithy analogy about black holes and Ippa's academic career.

Professor Jinu took a seat across from Ippa and looked her over carefully, as if Ippa was a newly arrived specimen for the biblioplaza. Ippa had been just another student floating at the edge of Jinu's vision. The professor dealt only with the really great and the poor. Now she was dealing with Ippa.

She finally spoke, "When you first came, there was doubt among the faculty." She paused to put her hands behind her back. "Your race is not known for their prowess of research and complex thought. However, your performance at first was a pleasant surprise."

"Professor—"

"Do not talk. I have heard it all before." Jinu tilted her head, looking every inch an academic.

Ippa closed her mouth. She needed to sit through this, go back to her studies, and demonstrate that she heard Jinu's speech. Sincerely understood the discipline and accepted the message. She struggled to sit up straight in the sling chair.

"You were one of four students in your class to achieve Zenith on your entry test. It was most impressive. With high expectations, some of the professors started giving you slightly more difficult assignments to elevate your studies."

Ippa was confused and tried to neutralize her expression. "I've received the same work assignments as the other students."

"You completed the same assignments but with more difficult content."

Ippa remembered how annoyed she was when she had to dissect a tarnieo with three hearts when other Level Ones received a simple rodent carcass.

Jinu broke through Ippa's thoughts. "I assigned you Earth because it's a relatively unknown planet. You already knew enough about more renowned ones and this was a chance for you to prove yourself."

Professor Jinu performed a series of hand motions and Ippa's records appeared on the wall screen. Though Ippa knew what they would show, she dreaded their appearance. The numbers started out strong, dipped at the midpoint of Level One, raised slightly, and then plummeted.

"We don't have time to invest in someone who will not be able to keep up. And that idiosyncratic presentation you gave is a clear indicator you're not keeping up." Jinu clipped her words at the end.

Ippa leaned forward to speak, to defend herself, to change where this was going, but the professor shook her head.

"You had a commendable start. Now other professors have dwindled your assignments to the easiest in class, and still you are struggling. I do not think it is your fault. Your kind may simply not have the resilience needed for Shou University. I had high hopes for you. You may not believe this…but this is difficult for me too.

"You're released from the university."

Cold despair washed over Ippa, her entire future black. Even the revelation that one of the strictest professors at The Shou had been impressed by her work, a comment that any other day would have lifted Ippa's entire outlook on life, was worthless now. Even worse, it was meaningless.

Ippa's mouth was dry, but she fought to speak. "I can do it—I can catch up."

"Ippa, you're not suited for university life. For all the intention behind the application process and entrance exams, sometimes this happens. You were pacing well, but you are no longer able to keep up.

We can't devote any more academic attention to you."

Ippa needed Jinu to see. "I could t-take a break. I could go at a slower pace."

"No, Ippa. There is not enough time for those options."

Ippa was furious, finally more angry than scared. "You have as much time as there is in the crisping universe! The university has always been here, is always going to be here. Why can't I have more time?"

Professor Jinu was miffed by Ippa's words. "The fact that you don't understand is precisely why you cannot continue here."

# Chapter 3

## Planet No. 68,902

A group of creatures moves across the desert with difficulty. They are dwarfed by the spindly rock formations that scratch the clear, orange atmosphere. In the far distance, too far away to worry the group, swirling tornadoes of dust and sand race across the open desert. The creatures move upright on two legs but without finesse. One heavy step destabilizes the other. They are used to scaling the sides of cliffs and digging through caves. Crossing flat distances is exhausting work for them.

Two smaller creatures, young ones, lead a group of full-grown adults, five in number.

The previous night, after eons of pressure and an increasing level of brittleness, one of the tall rock formations collapsed upon itself. The thundering crack rang through the dark hours, waking everyone in the hamlet.

Already, memory of the event fades. In the morning, they know there was a change, but in the minds of the creatures, soon it will be as if the massive rocks always lay broken on the ground. If pressed, they could remember that once the rubble stood upright (it would only be logical), but they do not often remember.

The boys investigated the area first thing after waking a second time. Crossing the flat land is easier for them. They are impatient with their elders.

"Come, come, come you," one boy cries. He is excited the adults are listening and treating him like one of them, which he will be soon. A legless sand creature, the dull yet golden color of aged rock, keeps pace with the other child. As well as limbs, it has no eyes but not every pet needs such.

"Travel, travel I," a female responds.

They arrive at the jagged but open mouth. The boys are quick to use their developing upper bodies to clamber down. They look top-heavy but are not so unbalanced as the adults. The boys' armor is thinner and their legs are more flexible. They will shed into proper adults when the rains come.

A few paces behind, the adults follow suit and descend. The creatures' arms are powerful. They need to be, for the amount of climbing and digging they do. Their thick exoskeleton protects them from falling rocks and keeps them cool from the sun. The heavy shell is dotted with bristles to help them feel their way through tight caves. The largest platelets stretch across the arms and legs while an intricate knitwork covers the abdomen and torso. At the joints and stomach, wherever platelets end by necessity of movement, thick, sandy-colored hide peers through.

The sand creature descends last, its strong abdominal muscles, tough scales, and resilient body make up for lack of limbs. It does well enough climbing down, until it is too steep. The sand creature sucks in its more delicate feelers, rolls into a ball, and lets gravity bring it down to the floor of the cave.

"Look you," one boy says to an adult.

"Look, see, hear all," the other young says and goes to check his pet.

The adults click with laughter at the boys' enthusiasm. The adults do not normally approve of the insistent vocal tone, but today they chuckle, indulgent.

It is a good, open space. Deep underground like it is, it could be used as a cool storage area for foodstuffs or a safe house when the biggest sandstorms come. Possibly a meeting space for large ceremonial gatherings, ones that should take place under the shelter of rock for proper reverence, though it would be hard for the oldest of them to reach on foot.

"Use?" one of them finally asks. It is not a light question. Though the word comes out toneless, the others know it is fraught with implications and unknowns. It is new. It is untried.

It is too good to pass up.

"Use we."

"Use we."

"Take we." Everyone is in agreement.

The group scatters to explore the new space so they can bring back word to their hamlet. The final decision will be made as a community, but this group will have to provide exhaustive details.

A male creature explores farther in than the boys. Out in the open plains, his gait was interrupted. He lets the memory fall away, leaving his brain to focus on the current moment. Instead of walking on two legs, he scales the cavern side and claws across, climbing in some areas, swinging across others. Despite the bulk of his armor, he moves gracefully. He does not scratch or break rock unless he wants to. He moves through two chambers, noting rock formations.

He comes to a third chamber, dark enough to interfere with his vision. A thickened ridge shades his eyes from the harsh sun, but it makes sight difficult deep in the rock. He takes a crystal out of an arm pouch their sort has evolved over time and blows on it. The crystal blooms with rose-colored light, stimulated by the exhale of carbon dioxide.

He continues until the tiny pads on his snout flame with sensation. His sight may be severely limited in the dark but short bristles along his back and arms as well as a highly sensitive snout make up for it. He perceives extreme moisture. There is a weak spot in the ground and he makes his way to it. It is short work to break the rock. He listens precisely as the wreckage falls and lands on more stone. He takes his time as he descends, uncertain what is below. A rush of movement catches his attention. If this is an underground stream, he would do well to keep out of the water. His heavy body cannot swim. The idea has never occurred to him and opportunity has never presented itself on the dry planet.

He blows on the crystal again and holds it high above his head. The first thing he notices is a narrow but deep underground river. It is only as wide as his height. From where he crouches, he knows it is very cold.

The new source of water will be a pleasant surprise for their community. Though the spring is located a substantial distance from the hamlet, the water may be useful for traveling or working groups.

Something catches his eye. A shape bobs along in the water. Many shapes.

The idea of harnessing the momentum and buoyancy of water to move something is not a common thought on his planet, but he is intelligent. It is obvious the items were intentionally placed in the water. Or rather, he sees them and feels the intention. The abstract past action eludes him.

Therein, he quickly understands the danger. Someone else knows about the underground river and uses it. Their kind is territorial, as much as they can be when hamlets are located so far apart.

He considers telling the young not to come back to this place, but it is too intriguing. He reaches out a long arm and halts one of the parcels. He struggles to lift it out of the water, but eventually he gets the item onto dry rock. It is hard and completely smooth, made from a substance he has never encountered before. He lightly runs his hands along the sides of it and lifts it close to his nose to smell carefully. The scent sets his determination to get inside. There's an apparatus to open the parcel, but his digits are not dexterous enough to operate it. He casually smashes it.

Among thin air pockets encased in slippery, smooth sheets is a lumpy, bound bag. Yes, juicy root vegetables. The root vegetable does not have a specific name in his language. More of a tone, an inflection to the societies' word for *eat*.

His stomach rumbles and his mouth goes wet. He has not eaten these juicy foods in a long, long time, but he also senses danger in his sides. Someone bundled this food carefully. Territorial displays or outright attacks are not unheard of when it comes to food or water possession in the desert. And this food is rare.

Cautiously, he looks through the holes on either side where water rushes in and out. Then, he cannot help it. He breaks the root with his widely splayed digits and horny nails. Evolution dictated his type have dangerous talons for fighting and climbing, but his fingernails are cut neatly—a sign of his civility and secure placement in a hamlet.

He chews and reaches for another handful. He cannot help it. Although he knows there is an ownership of the food by someone else, it is intangible.

He gorges himself and finishes one bag, yet he cannot believe it is gone already and reaches for another item, bobbing in the stream.

He is disappointed. Instead of food, there is a small sack of glossy black rocks and light, dried grass. Neither rare nor common, he wonders why someone would bundle those rocks. They are not good for toolmaking. The grass though could be useful. It grows sporadically across the desert.

As he climbs up and away toward the main chamber, he cannot believe what he found. Movement of water transporting items. And root vegetables.

Who do they belong to?

The taste in his mouth turns sour and, suddenly, he wishes they did not know of this place.

He goes to the group and says, "Go, go we." The urgency in his voice startles everyone and they climb upward, toward the shafts of hot light. The boys each carry one end of the sand snake. They are slower climbing up than when they went down.

The unknown scares him. He has trouble articulating what he saw to the others.

"Go water. Go eat. Eat I." He thinks and adds another "go" in an ominous tone.

His mind tires from thinking about what he saw under the ground. As visiting the cave is not yet habit, the memory threatens to slip away, but he brings it forward in his mind again and again. It is wild and distant. His brain would willingly let the incident disappear, but there is too much potential value. And much risk to assess.

He decides the supplies could only be going to one of the two cities. One city holds the Ruler. The other city is centered around a huge mine. He has never been to either city but has heard the tales that have become a part of himself as much as his own arms. When tales are spoken at ceremony, the entire hamlet listens and receives knowledge as powerful as instinct itself.

His partner enters the hollowed-out space in the side of the cliff where he is, their home. Fresh claw marks stand out in the aged rock. He expanded the resting space himself when his partner told him she would soon have kits, their own young ones at last.

"Care," he says.

"Care you," she says. She picks up a handful of tough fibers and with steady movements brushes off the day's dirt. She looks like him in form and size but has wide dark grooves on her shoulders and misses one digit, severed by accident long ago. Her legs are short and her arms powerful. She has always been beautiful to him.

He stands from his work: painstaking manipulation of rock to create tools. His inner shoulders feel like rocks themselves. Shaping rocks into tools is hard for his large hands, but he is proud of his status as one so skilled.

In few words, he tells his partner what he saw, focusing more on what he feels in the present than what happened in the past. Already she has heard. No one is talking of anything else. She shakes her head and sits quietly, thinking on such a thing.

"Take us," she says hesitantly.

"Ruin us." It could bring trouble. They can't know the hidden consequences, if any.

"Take," she says smaller. It is a simple phrase, but the inflection says it all: a little will not be missed. And if it is, so what? Is another hamlet going to travel impossible distances over a few missing foodstuffs? She is more sensible than him. Many of the females in the hamlet are expecting kits. An unexpected source of food would do them well.

She blows on the largest of the rose stones. The sun has almost set.

He walks to the open rock facing out of the hamlet. The ground is death-defying far, but there is no threat of falling to him. The air is neither hot nor cold. There is no humidity. He has not seen clouds in nearly a decade, but he would figure they would be coming soon, if anyone knew how to ask him.

He thinks about the hungry kits that will soon arrive as he watches a sand creature blurring away from the settlement. They have not hatched yet, but already his care for them is like the brilliant blue crystals of the north. He will provide for them.

Their kind does not travel far distances. For any arrangement to happen between two communities utilizing the stream is unthinkable. However, all the leaders in the hamlet agree the packages must be going to one of the twin cities, both too far away to be a worry for that day. It is decided that they can take some of the food. It moves through their territory, so they have a right to a portion. They will leave enough so that those who are supposed to receive it may not notice any missing, or if they do, it will be ambiguous enough that they won't wish to fuss over a journey into another's home territory where they will have no advantage.

Sometimes when they go, there are no bundles in the water. Sometimes they carry rocks and strange supplies. Sometimes foodstuffs. The unwanted items from the bundles are left to lie on the cave floor, though a few are taken back to the hamlet as novelties. A stack of flat fibers, clean and white as the clouds. A long thin tube with melted sand on each end. An intricate weave of chain that is too small to haul things but too beautiful to leave.

Everyone is tense, waiting. They feel it coming.

The sky erupts above them. The rains arrive.

The moisture makes his platelets slide around too much, but he is happy for the water. It makes the plants abundant for a stretch. It is a time for celebration and relaxation. There will be many joining ceremonies and births.

He hides under an overhang. The rain will not stop for some time, but there is no hurry to get wet. He thinks fondly of his kits. They will come soon now. The extra food from the stream has come at a good time. The current young ones make a racket. It is the first time they have seen rain and it marks their last days as children. It is a drizzle, pattering onto the dry soil and rock.

He looks up. Something moves fast over the desert floor. Faster than a dust tornado. Alarm spreads through the community. Something is coming, something never seen before.

Did the rains summon terrible beasts as in the tales of old?

His mate descends the cliff face. Others climb down. For what, no one knows.

The thing rolls to a stop in front of the settlement. It sits, glaring; huge with skin shiny and hard—harder than his.

He trembles.

The sides of the beast open. Smaller beasts emerge, but they look nothing like the great one. Is it birthing its young in the season of rain? Are the newborns here to devour them, hungry in their earliest moments?

They are biped creatures, like him, and approach. They have shockingly small torsos and soft heads covered by a weak platelet. They chatter between themselves constantly. The amount of speech they use would have taken him days to create.

A creature of his own kind emerges from the beast. It is unmistakably one of his sort, only from another hamlet. Then he understands. There is no great beast. It is a vessel that moves.

He ignores the chattering beasts and focuses on the old one. It ambles along behind the strangelings that fan out around the hamlet members.

The older creature approaches. Rain splashes on his platelets. He accuses in an offhand but stern way, "Take you."

Everyone is uneasy. What does *this* have to do with *that*?

"Give taker. Punish taker."

The old one looks around, waiting.

One of those in the gathering points to him as the finder and first taker.

"Come taker." The old one turns away.

The strange beings move in toward him and he backs up as

quickly as he can. They speak rapidly and incomprehensibly.

His partner reaches out to push away the pests. They stand halfway up her chest. She swats at them.

One of the new beings raises a limb that is bigger than the other and there is a loud click. Something shoots out. She falls to the ground.

He expects her to get up, fine. How could something so small put her down on the ground?

She lays on the wet ground gasping, opening and closing her mouth wordlessly and rain pelts her head.

He smells it. The tangy brine of her precious orange blood seeping into the desert floor, mixing with the rain. Panic spreads. Some of his companions run up, others try to race across the cliff face.

He bellows and runs. He will smash the group. Little monsters that threaten her and the kits. He rages and thrashes close. He is hit by something small but with incredible force. Blood trickles out of his body. His life is over.

No. A powerful hum radiates through his body. He cannot move. He is lifted into the vehicle and life is dark.

# Chapter 4
## Yaniqui
### Agriculture Planet No. 4,278

Though the morning was dim, everyone in the labor camp was awake, preparing for the day. Rain had come in the night, breaking the insufferable heat wave. The damp cool air was a relief, but tiny midges hatched with the rainfall and peppered the air.

Yaniqui rolled on her waist wrap and went outside to pee in the dug shaft. Two midges flew up her nostrils and she swallowed at least one. She stood by the lodge's door and brushed her hair with a stiff comb while watching the sun rise. When she was younger, Maemi used a soft brush with a lacquer handle on her curls and dabbed perfumed oil on the inside bend of her arm. Just then, Maemi was sewing the edge of her stocking with a borrowed needle.

The humanoids around Yaniqui were family, but not friends. She and Maemi looked like the other humanoid aliens in that everyone was from somewhere else. The first time humanoids migrated across the galaxy, they were biologically the same, spawning from the same planet, one of the Original Nine that evolved Intelligent life. The other eight planets grew animoids, and none were as apt at conquering star systems as humans.

Over eons, humanoids were isolated into small population pockets by the galaxy-wide Peeling Sickness and the ancient celestial Black Wars. They interbred regionally and some populations lost the knowledge of interplanetary travel altogether. Others secreted their people away, awaiting safer times. Subspecies slowly grew off the stable trunk of humanity and evolved to fit the environmental trials of each new planet.

None of it concerned Yaniqui as much as the cloud of midges that hovered around her and Maemi as they walked. When the sun crested the horizon, the insects disappeared into the long shady grasses.

Yaniqui and her mother, possibly the last of their kind, had hardly sat to eat first meal when a teenage boy approached them. Maemi leaned forward attentively but waited for him to speak. The boy cleared his throat and said Fra Yu wanted to see Yaniqui Daful.

Yaniqui saw Maemi's breath catch in her throat. As law-abiding citizens (mostly), a summons to the regional overseer could mean only one thing: a notice about the scholarship application. And the answer wasn't a negative. Yaniqui's heart fluttered in panic. *This is it. This is the start.*

They hurried the rest of the food into their mouths so as not to waste anything, and brought the bowls back to Zimetta. Few looked curiously at them, but Yaniqui felt like she moved drunkenly as her brain whirled.

As they walked down the road, Maemi fluffed her hair in preparation of the meeting. She always fixed her hair before something important. Her curls remained thick and springy even as she aged, and fixing them was one of the few indulgences she had left. "Didn't I say the sunrise looked especially auspicious this morning?"

In fact, it looked like every other sunrise Yaniqui had seen the past ten years, but she didn't say anything that would dampen either of their spirits. Destiny was constant. Hope was rare.

Maemi approached Fra Yu's office door with dignity and knocked twice. She stood, shoulders tense, and Yaniqui looked around at the fields, both pretending to be patient. The door opened with a chime—Yaniqui had never been invited, so she was surprised that it did that no matter whether the door was locked or not. She quickly collected herself and tried to remove any guilt from her face as the Fra invited her in. Maemi waited outside, oblivious to her daughter's chronic burglary.

The smell of dust and plastic made the setting familiar until Yaniqui was awkwardly invited to sit in front of the overseer's desk. Until then, as a young, untroublesome worker, Yaniqui had had no cause to meet with Fra Yu. It struck Yaniqui that perhaps she had been called for another reason and she had a moment of panic.

"Well, Yanaqui," Fra Yu said, mispronouncing her name, "we've gotten word back—you've been selected in the academic lottery."

Yaniqui smiled. For the first time in years, there was news. There was something new in her life. And it was going to bring her closer to the fate she deserved.

"That's great—"

"But just because you were selected, doesn't mean you have to accept." Fra Yu folded his hands on top of a slight paunch, as if settling in for a long conversation.

Yaniqui tilted her head, trying to discern the meaning of the man's words. *Turn down the life-changing opportunity? Indeed.* She didn't even want the scholarship, but her eyes turned to slits. "Why wouldn't I? It's a good opportunity."

"Mmm-hmm, mmm-hmm, it could be." Fra Yu pulled at the fabric under one armpit. His face was dully contemplative, as if he had to decide for himself whether to go on a great voyage and improve himself, or stay on the labor planet. "Or it could not be."

Yaniqui hadn't expected fate to bring her to be questioned by a random man in an aged plastic chair. "What do you mean by that?" Yaniqui asked.

The overseer leaned back and folded his hands on his stomach again. "Well, often young people like yourself think they're going to have an adventure and everything is going to get better, but instead they dig themselves into a hole."

Yaniqui licked her lips. She wanted to tell this man she was leaving 4,278 and would never look back, but she spoke cautiously enough. "I think the idea behind the academic program is to equip people for a better standard of living."

There was no response and Yaniqui knew Fra Yu sensed the underlayer of snark.

"No, I understand," he said slowly, to make it clear he understood in theory why someone might entertain the idea of leaving the labor planet. "People your age believe they're going to live a life different than their parents. But the fact of the matter is, everyone here came because they lost something. And once that loss is a part of a family's story, it takes generations to climb out." He leaned forward. "Yaniqui, do you realize, if you leave to go to school, you're saddling your mother with both of your debt payments while you study?"

Yaniqui chose a spot on the wall to stare at. The manila paint was obviously two coats over brown but done poorly both times. The walls looked like smooth, ground meal with husks in it.

"Debt?"

Fra Yu nodded. "Sure. The cost of shipping you to this planet...the price of food and supplies over the past..." He paused to pull out the same Loscroll Yaniqui had swiped from his desk numerous times. He opened it, typed something, and turned it to face Yaniqui.

The floating numbers made Yaniqui dizzy. She knew there was debt—there was always debt for indentured laborers—but Maemi organized their abstract finances. To Yaniqui, they were insignificant numbers that would one day whisk away when destiny chose to act.

The overseer put the Loscroll away. "I'm just making you aware. You can stay here, work off your debt, save a little, and go to school later."

In the aftermath of their planet's death, Maemi had brought Yaniqui to 4,278 to hide. Their way of life was gone. Their beloved, Domi, who was on-planet at the time, gone. Their wealth was gone. Maemi's brilliant career and lavish lifestyle, gone. With no protection, and a lure that would bring the most powerful in the galaxy after them, Maemi thought it was better to hide as peasants under labor contracts than to be stolen, coerced, and trafficked to a fate no one could predict.

But along the way, the ruse that they were impoverished Parentheite refugees instead of gifted Wea Saavians protected by fate felt more and more like reality. A dim reality with a lackluster end.

The numbers changed nothing. Once she completed the mission her entire life had been building toward, Yaniqui would come back and find a way to save Maemi too. She shook her head. "I'm going."

Fra Yu peered at her a moment more, then slid an envelope across the desk. Yaniqui softly laid two fingers on it. It had been months since Yaniqui had held real paper, and that only a scrap of a glossy magazine passed from one young person to another through the flat grass seas of 4,278. The envelope was not thick, but Yaniqui could almost imagine she felt the fibers.

Outside, Yaniqui handed the packet to her mother who walked a discreet ten paces from the overseer's office and reverently tore the envelope open. She muttered to herself, looking for the lines she had dreamed of.

"'Yaniqui Daful has been chosen to attend Nourish Industries Inc. College on scholarship under the basis of being a refugee.' Yani! This is amazing!"

Maemi shuffled through the papers looking for the departure date. "We'll have to trade for some new clothes. I suppose you should continue to pretend to be Parentheite…that's what I wrote on your application and anyway no one's ever questioned it."

If Maemi was happy, Yaniqui was blooming. Life was suddenly thrown into high contrast. She could see every polished rock, every thread of Maemi's waist wrap. The moment seemed to go on forever. She was going to do it. She had paid her penance and now it was time for her to live. Fate had given her a way.

She'd been planning for months, hoping—almost knowing—that the big moment would come. Once she was off-planet, she'd ditch the plans to attend a crappy corporation-funded tech school and escape into the galaxy. Hloban was out there, somewhere. Her betrothed.

She was going to find him. Fate would lead the way.

But first.

"Maemi, Fra Yu told me about the debts."

Maemi looked across the fields as they walked. "It will work out. And honestly, what else could happen to us? We already live and work as slaves."

Yaniqui shook her head, exasperated. "We're not slaves. Things could be worse."

Maemi broke into a surprise smile that belied her words. "You're right, things can always get worse."

Yaniqui let out a rough sigh and turned away. Maemi was counting down the days to their discovery and eventual demise every time Yaniqui bothered to check. She had gone to such great lengths to keep their secret but still lived in fear. Something Yaniqui was not going to give in to.

Only on her home planet until she was an adolescent, Maemi's obsession with secrecy was a cultural struggle Yaniqui couldn't understand about her people. To have such a gift, such a belief in fate but also be scared about crisping everything.

Wea Saa had been an isolationist state by choice. The need placed upon them by other peoples and the Joint Council was constant and unbearable. Everyone wanted to be healed and only Wea Saavian women could heal them. Men could heal themselves, but just as they couldn't create life on their own, neither could they save one. Not like that.

Even in the days Wea Saa tried, they could never heal enough. Instead, Wea Saavians were kidnapped, taken so that healing went only to the most wealthy and powerful. So, her people turned inward, refused to heal, defended their air space, and were gradually left alone. But Wea Saavians were at risk any time they left Wea Saa. And Maemi and Yaniqui were utterly alone.

Or that's how Maemi would describe it. Yaniqui would—and had—argued that this was not the life meant for them. Fate would protect them if they would be bold enough to follow.

Now that she was accepted to school, the course of her life would shift by degrees. She would not have to dig and hide in the dirt. She would have opportunity and freedom. She could find Hloban.

Maemi's dream was for Yaniqui to get an education that would give her a safer life. Live better, yes, but also *hide* better. Yaniqui's dream was to find the fire in her life. To have what her parents had and what her grandparents had—their destiny. To her, it was a simple matter. It was the way of Wea Saa. Of course, she would find the one she was meant to be with. The placement of the stars at each of their births dictated they be together. If the stars mandated that they be together, the stars would help them find each other.

Yaniqui turned back to Maemi. "I'm sorry to leave you behind," she said shyly.

Maemi reached over and put her arm around Yaniqui's shoulders—a rare hug.

"What I dream of—what I've always dreamed of—is for you to have a better life. This is the way."

When Yaniqui was younger, she used to go with Maemi to fix satellites in the far reaches of their zone. Yaniqui had served Domi too as an early apprentice. Her parents took pride in her ability to support the community at such a young age.

The last time they went together, being with Maemi had saved her life.

Yaniqui was pretending to nap in the miniscule craft. Even as a Wea Saavian, her menstrual cycle still brought cramping. Yaniqui didn't wake up because she wasn't really asleep, but her mind snapped to attention when she heard the urgency in Maemi's voice. Maemi was frantically trying every channel to get through to Domi, her office, the emergency channel, anyone.

Yaniqui distinctly remembered jumping down from her bunk, free-falling, cushioned by the lack of gravity in the maintenance craft. Maemi turned, her eyes wide. "The sensors picked up an enormous amount of radiation."

"What? Where?"

Maemi fought to get out the words. "Near Wea Saa."

For days they had thought Wea Saa had been attacked. They shut down everything they could, drifted through space, only risking sending out signals every few hours before changing locations.

They finally learned what happened—a solar flare had struck out in the direction of Wea Saa. There was little warning as radiation rained down on their planet. In the span of a day, Yaniqui and Maemi lost their family, their culture, their world, and their future.

They were saved because they were off-planet.

So was Hloban.

He had been off-planet for his own apprenticeship and Yaniqui just knew Hloban had to be alive. However, the early work Maemi put into locating him brought about only false leads. In Maemi's eyes, he was either dead or unfindable in the enormity of the galaxy, which was as good as dead to her.

Of course, Yaniqui was irrevocably impacted by the loss, but her memories of Wea Saa faded with the years and she adapted quicker than Maemi to life on 4,278. As the mother, it was Maemi who lay awake at night wondering if their next second could be their last. If a catastrophic event was already racing through space to exterminate her daughter and reason for being. If news of who they were had already traveled to Akar. It was Maemi who worked so hard to keep them together.

Yaniqui's smile faltered. "What if you're transferred to another work site? What if I can't find you…after."

"You'll be in school. *I'll* find *you*."

Yaniqui swallowed hard. Yaniqui had always assumed Hloban would find her, but now, with the acceptance, Yaniqui would have a way out. She could escape and disappear among the stars. It was time for her to find him. And then, she would return. To rescue Maemi.

Word of the acceptance and scholarship traveled fast. More than ten people came up to congratulate Yaniqui at dinner that night. She flushed each time. Yaniqui had always been more outgoing than Maemi would have liked, but rarely did she have something worth her own pride.

Zimetta's youngest came with a second serving sent by the cook herself, nearly unheard of. Yaniqui looked at the bowl half-filled with the pasty mash. She had left many, many mealtimes not totally whole, but never once did she wish for more of *that*.

"I don't know why Mama's giving this to *you*. You'll be eating university food soon enough," Kimi said, her cheeks wobbling through a carefully placed frown.

Kimi was five years Yaniqui's junior, barely an adult herself, but Yaniqui rarely found it within herself to act benevolently towards the assistant cook. It was a good thing fate shone on her the way it did that day.

"Thanks, Kimi," Yaniqui said and smiled as if she were truly touched by the extra food. She said loudly, "I'll think of you every time I eat at the university cafeteria." Which would be not even a single time.

Maemi beamed and Yaniqui was pleased she tricked her mother into thinking her adult daughter was finally maturing at last.

Yaniqui took an obligatory spoonful and caught the eye of the young Vertruvian with the name of a whistle. She motioned for the little girl to come closer.

Yaniqui lowered her voice. "You'll need this for your recovery."

"Oh no, ma'am. I'm quite well." Despite her words, the girl took the food eagerly and Yaniqui was pleased to see she supported the bowl with both hands.

"Then share it with your siblings."

It felt nice to have something to give, and even nicer to have talked with so many as the stars arrived in the sky. Though Yaniqui didn't plan to set foot on campus—or if she did, just for a few days to get her bearings—she played her part. Every time someone asked how very thrilled was she to be going to school, Yaniqui thought of what she could remember of Hloban's face and let that fuel her excitement.

It seemed the only person that didn't come talk to Yaniqui was Sario. They didn't often eat meals together, Maemi being the way she was, but it would have been entirely appropriate for a friend to congratulate another on such good news.

She looked in his direction where he sat with his uncle and two older women, both, Yaniqui knew, had been born in the labor camp. She burned a hole in Sario's neck, but he didn't turn.

A shout came from one of the paths. Everyone looked. Roh leaned forward in interest and a few people stood to see better. A man entered the clearing, a woman shrinking at his side. He carried a large sack. No, Yaniqui realized, it wasn't a sack or a bundle of clothes, it was a young boy. The woman held a fistful of rags to the boy's neck, obscuring his face.

Bowls sat untouched as the crowd gawked at the newcomers. As they took in the distraught trio, an ominous air washed over the crowd.

The man looked over the heads of the seated people. He opened his mouth and his voice cracked. He swallowed hard, his chest heaving, and tried again. "We're looking for the healer."

Everyone glanced around as if a talented healer would appear, but the infirmary was a good walk away.

"We're looking for Yaniqui."

Next to Yaniqui, Maemi's shoulders went tense. Her mouth drew down as if it were suddenly made from granite.

Yaniqui herself was shocked. The only person who knew was Sario. She swiveled her head to find her oldest friend. They made eye contact. His eyes were wide, a mirror image of her own, but from guilt, not surprise.

Zimetta was pointing the couple and their wounded child in the direction of Yaniqui, but with a confused look on her face. "She's just a field hand. You need to get to the infirmary!" she yelled to their backs.

The man dropped to his knees in front of Yaniqui. Everything disappeared except the boy's ashen face. A scarlet swirl spoiled the cloth at his neck. Yaniqui knew the man was yelling, but she couldn't hear him. Someone—Maemi, urging her to go?—pulled at her shoulder.

Though Yaniqui had never feared discovery the way Maemi had, she had never been stuck between immediate, public exposure and someone's fast-approaching death.

The woman grabbed at Yaniqui's hand and tried to force it toward her son. Maemi flung her bowl aside. Maemi and the other mother pushed and shrieked at each other while a mass of people shouted advice.

Then Sario was at Yaniqui's side. The man shouted at him, but his mouth was so full of sorrow she could hardly understand.

"Oh crisps, Yani. This is my cousin and her husband. Their sites run parallel to ours. This is their kid. You've gotta save him!"

Once again, every face turned toward Yaniqui. Everyone in the camp understood Sario knew Yaniqui best.

She turned dagger eyes on him, her voice suddenly gone.

He hit her shoulder with the back of his hand. "The kid is going to bleed out," he shouted over the noise of the crowd.

It was true. The boy was in a bad way. She was furious with Sario—this could disrupt everything—but she couldn't let this boy die in front of her.

Yaniqui shook herself. She didn't look at Maemi, couldn't look at her. Her hands rose like they were born to. Yaniqui jerked the wet cloth aside. She saw a few ragged stitches of thread in the meat of the neck, holding enough blood in to stave off death but doing nothing to fix the deep damage. The father howled, but already Yaniqui had her hands against the boy's neck, staunching the blood.

Her hands warmed, not from the blood, but from the energy her own body was expelling. She felt the jaggedness of broken skin and ripped muscle deep within herself. It was as if her own body was shredded, as if her own neck was ripped. Her collarbones felt white-hot. Yaniqui imagined the pieces knitting together, felt a small relief in her own neck. The lifeblood of the boy pulsed more slowly over her hands, but still it came.

Tears dripped down Yaniqui's face in pain and frustration. She never had to heal such a deep wound so quickly. The back of her neck went damp with effort.

The boy was going to die. Yaniqui couldn't do it.

Suddenly another hand pressed on the side of the boy's neck. Yaniqui looked up with a start. It was Maemi, the corner of one black eye trained on Yaniqui. But she looked resolute. The healing quickened and Yaniqui's body calmed.

Shaking, she pulled her sticky hands from the boy's neck. It was still smeared with blood, but it looked raw rather than hacked to pieces. The thread burrowed into his now knitted skin. Yaniqui struggled to pinch it with her slick fingers. When she got it at last, she tugged gently, but the skin would not give it up.

Blood thrummed in her ears. She was weak with exertion. And she would rather have a dragon soar out of the sky and engulf her in fire than turn to face Maemi. She asked the only question she could make sense of. "What happened to him?"

The mother took a long sniff and wiped her nose on her sleeve. "A rock went through the chipper. Shrapnel struck him just after the last break."

Maemi turned to Sario with a question of her own. "What have you done?"

# Chapter 5

Hloban (*ł-o-ben*)
New Washington, WI, Earth

Hloban sat outside the view of the camera. He was a consultant, not the main attraction.

Secretary-General Cortez sat stiffly, waiting. A page came and whispered something in her ear. She nodded back and put her fingerprint on a virtual document. The secretary-general of the United Nations once again corrected her posture and waited, looking at the camera as if she had nothing better to do than be long-sufferingly attentive to a blank screen. Hloban could tell from the indignation of the aids this was not a woman who often waited.

Hloban didn't like waiting either, but these sessions were always the same—full of dead time. It took him weeks of talking the secretary-general's office through the larger framework of their communications strategy (and where they could be misunderstood or accidently cause offense), then the specifics of arranging the meeting between on- and off-planet participants, and finally review Cortez and her staff on expected etiquette. After all that work, it still all came down to waiting. The technology was ready. The Earthlings were in their places. But

Joint Council members worked on their own schedules, which did not necessarily abide by meeting start times.

Hloban quite liked his own role though. That morning, he put on a rich caramel-colored suit and a crisp raspberry shirt. He thought the colors offset his short black hair nicely. As professional as he looked, Hloban wouldn't have any screen time. If he had a concern, he would signal Emmett, who would decide whether it was worth interrupting the secretary-general. Hloban's most excellent suit was merely for his benefit and those around him.

The screen flickered to life as an Earth satellite received the Interstellar Wave from Star Tau Ceti, the nearest transmitter twelve light-years away. Cortez further straightened in her chair as members of the Joint Council appeared.

Joint Council Members Deyo and Kilberg were just seating themselves in a bland meeting room across the galaxy. On their side of the screen, Kilberg waved away a cup of muna tea. Cortez looked to her page and nodded. Hloban was careful not to catch her eye as she turned back to the camera. He knew she wanted to look busy in front of those whom she considered her counterparts.

"Greetings Council Members Deyo and Kilberg."

Hloban picked up the emphasis on Kilberg's name.

Deyo responded, "Greetings, Earth United Nations Secretary-General Elia Cortez."

Cortez's mouth twisted in a smile. Days ago, Cortez grilled Hloban on why they couldn't just call her "Secretary-General Cortez."

"There's no other Secretary-General Cortez out there," she insisted. "Should I start calling them "Off-planet Joint Council Members Brian Deyo and Rezario Arsehole Kilberg?"

Hloban had smiled. "I'm not sure that's the name Kilberg's mother gave him, ma'am."

"Well, I'm sure I'm not alone in thinking it should have been."

Cortez, Kilberg, and Deyo continued the customary greetings of inquiring after each other's home planet and sighing over how busy they've all become in their work. Hloban shrugged at Emmett when their eyes met. This was how it was supposed to go. Emmett rolled his eyes back and tapped his wrist—something Hloban gathered

Earthlings did to signal the time, though after years on-planet, he wasn't sure why.

On his home planet, Wea Saa, Hloban had been a page himself in the ambassador's edifice. Those early years of fetching documents, making muna tea, and drafting basic correspondence meant that he was nearly the most experienced person on Earth when it came to communicating with the Joint Council (Jeb had him beat). His end-of-term page duties brought him to the Joint Council itself as a capstone to the training. His knowledge, which he had considered limited before arriving on Earth, was in high but unsteady demand on a planet trying to find its place in the politics of the larger galaxy.

Organizations and governments contracted him as an interpreter but not in language. He interpreted culture and societal norms for those pursuing business or diplomacy off-Earth. Hloban did his best to convince Earthling executives that though their counterparts from other planets were animoids, they had to give up that who's-a-good-doggie voice Earthlings unconsciously used with animals. He advised government officials not to reveal how much plastic was in their oceans—it only served to make everyone distrustful of them. He helped Earthlings navigate waters that were second nature to him.

"We've discussed it," Deyo was saying. "We appreciate Earth applying for voting membership—"

"—*again*, at the earliest possible allotment since the Joint Council's last response," Kilberg put in.

"But," Deyo continued, "Earth has not yet reached the point where it could be realistically considered an active participant in galaxy-wide proceedings. I believe the United Nations itself has its own permanent observer states?"

Cortez placed a careful smile on her face. "Yes, but they're not members of the United Nations like Earth is an accepted member of the Joint Council."

"This is true, but still not the way things are done at the Joint Council," Deyo said.

Emmett shot a glance at Hloban, who nodded. They both looked back to Cortez, but she was having a hard time interrupting Deyo's explanation that Earth wasn't ready to participate at the voting level.

The Joint Council was happy to connect Earth with information, and *someday* Earth would be given the opportunity to vote alongside the other planet members.

"Yes, but when?" Cortez demanded. "That is the exact same language I've heard the last two times. I'm looking for concrete information—" Cortez glanced in Hloban's direction, remembering the metaphor would make no sense to her counterparts "—rock-solid, that is. I want a solid answer."

Kilberg turned their mics off and turned to Deyo to confer.

Emmett snapped his fingers at Hloban, panicked. "Get up there," he mouthed at Hloban.

Cortez had shut off her own microphone by the time Hloban perched at her side.

"I don't know how I can be any more direct," she told Hloban. "I want an answer or I will keep requesting meetings." She wasn't expecting great counsel but wanted to look busy while complaining.

"Meetings that they have to take but only serve to waste your time and theirs, Secretary-General. They likely cannot give a straight answer. It's more of an organic process than you'd expect. If they gave the wrong time estimation, they'd feel terrible about providing you with incorrect information."

"I'm sure Kilberg is terrified of disappointing me," Cortez said dryly.

Suddenly, Kilberg spoke, mic back on, and Hloban couldn't help but double-check they didn't have a hot mic. No—safe.

Hloban stepped aside as Cortez switched herself on.

"Excuse me, Earth United Nations Secretary-General Elia Cortez, who was that being?"

Cortez couldn't help but glance at Hloban off-camera but covered her surprise. "A consultant."

"Could you bring him back?"

Everyone looked expectantly at Hloban. Appearing on-camera briefly while the conversation was paused was one thing. This? This made sweat break out on the back of Hloban's neck.

"Yes," Kilberg said when he spotted Hloban again. "I recognize you from the brief for this meeting. You're the Wea Saavian?"

"Yes, Council Member Kilberg."

"You may go." Kilberg waved him offscreen.

Hloban moved away, but his heart was frozen. To say the name of his people so casually, to strike him full of sorrow with such an offhanded remark; Hloban thought there might be something to Cortez's nickname for Kilberg.

"Secretary-General Cortez, we've noticed the number of refugees Earth has taken on of late." Kilberg spoke as if he wanted nothing more than to guide Earth through infanthood, but Hloban sensed a barb coming. Everyone did. The room was thick with tension at this unexpected and therefore unprepped topic. "Including high-profile cases like the Wea Saavian. Earth seems to have an interest in offering sanctuary to rare, endangered species. Especially those with such abilities. Which gives us cause for concern."

Cortez went red in the face. "Pardon me, Council Member Kilberg, we are not here today to discuss our refugee program. But since you inquired, yes, few other planets were willing to offer sanctuary to this man who lost his home planet. One of our values on Earth is that everyone who needs a home has a home."

Hloban winced. He didn't like being discussed in this manner, but more than that, he'd warned Cortez in the past not to gloss over Earth's transgressions. The Council would know. Already knew. They always did.

Kilberg nodded slowly. "Yes, a crucial value indeed. However, I caution Earth against trying to artificially inflate its influence."

"I beg your pardon?" Cortez kept her voice even, as he'd coached her. No point in looking like uneducated barbarians.

"We worry Earth is overstepping its role by trying to inflate the number of races represented on-planet in hopes of forcing action by the Joint Council regarding membership."

"That is," Deyo stepped in, "we know you are aware one of the requirements for voting membership is off-planet entries—evidence that immigration, trade, and education take place on a certain level. Is Earth perhaps trying to mimic those organic interactions by taking on refugees?"

Cortez shook her head. "I can state unequivocally that is not the case. Now, are you going to answer my question—" Hloban cringed when she said "you" instead of the representatives' titles "—or shall my office work on setting up the next meeting between the three of us?"

Deyo and Kilberg looked at each other, some silent conversation taking place.

"Like I said before," Deyo said, looking directly at Cortez, "becoming a voting member for the Joint Council is a complex process, the—"

"Give me an estimate of some kind. A standardized year? Three years? A decade?"

"Generations."

The word hung in the air.

Cortez inhaled deeply through her nose. "I appreciate your forthcoming answer. Thank you for your time, Joint Council Members Deyo and Kilberg."

The screen went dark. The secretary-general rose and stretched her back. Her attention was quickly consumed by a page, but she looked up long enough to thank Hloban. "It wasn't the answer we were looking for, but anyway, I'm sorry they involved you."

"Do not concern yourself at all, Secretary-General."

Hloban was dismissed with a nod and commiserated with Emmett briefly before starting the long process of exiting the United Nations headquarters and making his way home. Meetings with the Joint Council were always a rush, but he was reluctant about anything that would make him findable.

And though what Kilberg implied about the United Nations's desire to inflate Earth's numbers had a threat of truth to it, it wasn't any of his business.

Hloban believed in self-invitation. After all, he was on Earth and how would he have gotten there if he didn't ask himself in?

But he still felt like he had to invite himself into his own home. If Hloban had gotten a flash of this unexpected future as a child, the ordinary act of arriving home would have astonished him. A bathroom door was off the eating area—gross—and, speaking of which, the eating area wasn't even outside. The walls didn't reconfigure via verbal command. Music played on invisible speakers that Hloban had been excited about until he discovered they were merely hidden pieces of plastic, not invisible after all. The music itself was Earthling.

And Loera.

At the counter, his wife drank a glass of cucumber water while writing in her planner (she preferred paper for home life, digital at work). She looked up and smiled. No one was warmer or more genuine than she was. Hloban's black hair was only light by comparison to her jet twist out, but in that moment, a stray ray of sunshine lit up the curly hairs along the tips.

Hloban originally wanted to live closer to the center of New Washington where both the U.S. government and the U.N. operated out of, but Loera insisted on a child-friendly neighborhood and because of his status as an expatriate, they were limited in selection. Whenever Hloban made a positive comment about the new capital, New Washington, Wisconsin, every Earthling within hearing distance lamented the loss of the old capital. Their sacred monuments entrenched in the sea. The old White House that was actually white. Hloban didn't get all the particulars, but he had to bite his tongue from suggesting that they shouldn't have melted their polar ice caps. But what did he know? He didn't even have a planet anymore.

He leaned in to kiss Loera's cheek while handing her a woven bag and was rewarded with the clean scent of fresh cucumber. He got out his own cup for a glass of juice as Loera pulled out a wooden train and track set from his bag.

"I thought I told you," she said, "I picked up Obani's birthday present earlier this week. The new animatronics? They're tiny, but a set was as expensive as my first paycheck." Loera tucked the toy back in the bag. "They're going to be a hit though. Didn't I tell you, Hoban?"

Hloban did not hear the mispronunciation of his name anymore. Or hardly did.

"Yeah, but I wanted to pick out a gift too." Hloban put the juice back in the fridge. "I think I'll take Obani to the library and get a book on trains," Hloban said.

Loera looked away, too casually. She adjusted her glasses.

Hloban put his drink down on the counter but kept a grip on it. She didn't even have to say anything. He could sense it. "What, Loera?"

Loera looked a little guilty now. "I'm not saying it's a big deal."

"What? Tell me," Hloban said in a rush. "Is the train set inappropriate? Is it against social norms to gift one except in the month of February, during the leap year? Were these devices used to cart prostitutes across North America? Are they associated with drugs? What is so wrong with the present I picked out?"

"Nothing, nothing," Loera said. She paused. The kitchen wall ticker relayed the weather and an update on a company Loera was tracking news alerts on. Her eyes darted toward the ticker but she said, "They're kind of considered an old-person gift. You know, something your great-aunt might get you. Wooden toys are very old-fashioned."

Hloban drank his juice. He caught the swing of Loera's earrings as she covertly peeked at his face to see if he was offended, which made him drink his juice longer. It was petty, and if he drank any more of the sweet drink, he'd be sick, but he couldn't help it.

He finally put his glass down, licked his top lip, and decided to neutralize everything. "It'll be fine. I'll play trains with him. I think he'll like it." It was conspicuously quiet. "Where is Obani?"

"My mom took him to the play park. I thought it'd be nice to have some peace at home."

Hloban nodded. Loera's job was more intense than his. As an alien, he was not permitted to take any job from an Earthling. And she, well, everyone wanted Loera's golden touch on their projects.

She was partner at an enormous lab that produced antimatter fuel. Loera spent little time in the sterile lab itself these days. Instead, she focused her efforts on the unrelenting progression of operations and mentored several young people with their own start-ups. Hloban was proud that her vision and energy propelled the experimental research center into a prospering company. It also meant that at home, she valued things like quiet time when Hloban's own schedule was nearly all quiet time peppered with random consulting jobs.

Hloban made a snack (thinly sliced kohlrabi with tiny sardines and a light sauce on top, the closest thing he could get to a dish he grew up with, one Loera would never try) while Loera described Obani's preschool friend, Steph. Her mother said that she could not have animal products or refined sugar and to watch her at the birthday party because she'd taken to raiding others' pantries, stuffing sweets in her socks.

"I should add something to the menu for her. Or maybe Steph's mom would like you to cook for her," Loera said, eyeing Hloban as he took another bite. Loera hurried the conversation along.

Hloban knew she wanted to put the insult she'd dealt about the wooden train many words behind them.

Loera closed her planner and drifted over to Hloban. He wasn't mad. Even after six years together, they still communicated differently from entirely different perspectives. At one of Loera's benefit events, an American with a husband from another country tried to empathize about cross-cultural mishaps in relationships, but it was entirely different than when people grew up on different planets. Countries? Those were neighbors. Hloban privately thought the man was just an asshole for not offering to celebrate cultural holidays with his husband.

Hloban finished chewing and drank the rest of his juice. He didn't care about the train or the party menu anyway.

He put one hand on Loera's waist under her blazer and slipped it under the band of her pants. She was warm through her tucked-in shirt. He ran his other hand up the smooth nape of her neck. Loera leaned into Hloban and everything else was gone. He wasn't breathless or dizzy, but entrenched in the puzzle of how to unbutton her shirt in the smoothest way.

He kissed her and wondered if his mouth tasted like fruit or fish. Her tongue was hot on his. Loera pulled on Hloban's shirt with one hand and ran her fingers through his dark hair with the other. Thank the gods it was fruit. He let out a soft noise.

Hloban made up his mind to set Loera on the counter and start with a button or two and nuzzle his face into new territory.

She pulled away, "Oh no, I forgot to confirm the delivery time of the 3-D simulation for the party." Loera dashed to her planner and rifled through the pages.

Hloban straightened his shirt. He thought the cost of the simulator was over the top for a kid's party and had offered to host Obani's friends in his own spacecraft—nothing could beat the real thing, right?—but Loera wondered where everyone would sit for cake.

The moment was gone. "I'm going to check my messages. If you want me to express an order of those little cabbages for that kid, let me know," Hloban said.

"Brussels sprouts," Loera called behind him.

Hloban went upstairs into the home office. He heard Loera turn on her video communicator as he shut the door. He did not lock the door. That was key to feeling guilt-free.

The wall console sprang to life when he looked at it. It stretched a full wall, half viewer for images with a dozen icons and tickers on the lower half. It was Earth-made but Hloban took out a small gray device from a bin on the top shelf of the closet that was not locked. Hloban told himself many times that because it could be accessed by anyone in the household, it was not classified as hiding. Though it was doubtful that Loera would search through a bin of old appliance warranties and manuals.

Loera's office had an interstellar drive like this one. It was too expensive for every household to have one, but Hloban bought one from Jeb because they weren't every household.

To Hloban, receiving wireless signals in seconds from a transmitter in another star system was standard. He thought it was cute when Earthlings expressed their bewilderment. Everyone accepted the antimatter fuel and negative matter entries that allowed for faster-than-light speed travel, but for a signal to travel that sort of distance in seconds? Hloban always began by explaining how the big bang expanded the universe faster than light speed but around sentence two attentions waivered.

Hloban typed in the address for an interstellar nongovernmental missing person's message board. The newest notices appeared and he skimmed them automatically.

A baby found abandoned in a large shopping center. No genetic tests done yet. Currently with a religious organization.

Two girls found dead with puncture wounds in the sides of their necks. Physical descriptions and contact information for sector officiants followed.

Information on an uncouth animoid found living in an off-planet parking area and a plea for someone to please come and remove it.

Hloban filtered the search criteria. It took eight minutes to sift through the results. There was nothing for him there.

He visited the Interplanetary Endangered Races Resource (IERR). Nothing new so Hloban continued down his usual list of places to check.

There was no indication that any other Wea Saavian had been found, no notices that any of his people still existed out in the galaxy. He didn't expect any change a decade after his planet died but continuing to search was like holding a very long wake. And once he stopped, his tribe would be truly dead.

Finally—and this was the part that made his heart speed—he entered Yaniqui Daful's missing person's code (000620112520133) to see if anything came up.

It didn't.

He would continue to hold wake for her the rest of his life. It was his responsibility, the only thing he could do to keep the memory alive of a funny, scrawny girl he had been betrothed to in another life.

Hloban erased the log and pulled up the results for a sports match. He quickly clicked through a few other go-to sites on Earth's internet to create an explainable and realistic history and memorized the outcome of a game he heard about that morning. It was difficult identifying why he went to such great lengths to hide his ritual from Loera, but one reason was that he felt ungrateful while he did it. As if he didn't appreciate the second chance at life he had, or that he was too fixated on a past that should have been his future.

There was a sudden crash downstairs. Hloban flew to the office door, but when he heard Loera laugh, he slowed. In the kitchen he found her sprawled on the floor, righting herself.

"I fell, but I saved the cake," she said.

Hloban smiled and pushed the baked but unfrosted cake farther onto the counter, where it would be safe. There was a gouge in one side.

"We can fill the hole with frosting. That will be my piece," Loera said. She slipped off her blazer. "Hey, want to join me down here?"

# Chapter 6

## In Transit

When he wakes, his vision is filled with new things. The vehicle bumps along and makes noises he has never heard before as it grinds sand and broken stone. Rain patters on the top. His torso and ankles are bound with something harder than rock. He is sitting up at least but can hardly move.

Some of the weird creatures had removed their protective platelets and he feels disgust when he sees how slender and weak their bodies are. They have puny shoulders and their neck is open and unprotected. He can even see their lifeblood pulse. How could *this* enemy take him down? His brain flashes an image of a small but poisonous scorpion, but the comparison doesn't feel right.

He thrashes and bellows, but he cannot move because of the restraints. He presses hard against the binders. It pulses a fearsome shock into him like the rare, blue-hot lightning of the rains.

"Release." He tries to engage the old creature, but is resolutely ignored. He speaks again and again, but the old one won't look in his direction. Won't explain anything. He knows he was taken because of the resources, but why? And why did they not confront him there, at the stream, so all could understand without many words? Instead, they came to his hamlet and captured him.

He wonders about his mate. The memory of her falling threatens to slip away, but he brings the sight to mind again and again. Is she alive? Are she and the kits dead?

He expects to be taken to one of the twin cities. He sees one of them—he is not sure which—in the distance as they drive by. A grey mist obscures an immense mountainside of homes. Even close enough to see, it would take him days to walk there on his own legs. The vehicle turns in a different direction.

The smaller beings chatter relentlessly. He bellows occasionally. He sleeps after a time, but it is fitful and unsettled.

A greater level of commotion wakes him as the small creatures make noise putting their platelets back over their heads, unfastening rope-like harnesses that hold them into place. The door opens and his nasal pads flare at the new air. The old one is the first out and moves staggeringly across the ground. Three beings block his view and he can tell they are worried to get too close to him for they chatter a long, long time before one connects a metal stick to his wrist fastenings. They unbind his feet and he kicks out. His legs are not the strongest part of him, but all he needs is to push them away and maneuver himself out. Instead, electric fire shocks him. It takes another shock before he lets himself be led along like a dumb beast.

The vehicle drives away and it is only a few steps through the rain to a structure. The creatures did not hollow out a cave like his kind but carved and stacked rocks to build cavern walls. It looks strange standing upright in the otherwise empty landscape. There's a smattering of other buildings close by, all with strips of metal up to just above where he could jump. He desires to climb and tear down the walls in a rage. A buzz of electricity runs through the metals. His rage is useless.

The creatures bring him into the building through an evenly cut door with smooth, flat sides. He feels uneasy entering this artificial place. His captors guide him through a series of rooms with more of the odd creatures. They chatter and chatter. A few look up at him. He moves carefully to avoid being zapped again. The old one is nowhere.

He panics when they bring him at last to a room with bindings on the floor. A creature jabs him in the side with an electric zapper. He thinks he is dying now, finally now. He bellows, but it fades away and he comes to on the ground, bound across and around all his limbs and his torso.

A voice enters the room. He cannot swivel his head to see because of thick blinders on either side.

"Yosef, get moving. I don't want more paperwork because you're late on this."

Someone turns the dials of a contraption. It is fire and heat lightning, but he cannot get away.

With a strong hiss, it burrows into his chest platelet. He never imagined something hurting him there, the strongest part of him. He roars without words.

The man hurting him ignores his reaction. "Is it a male or female?"

A woman murmurs something and someone else says, "Male."

He looks down at his shoulder, reliving the pain when he sees the strange marks left upon his armor.

"D-68," a voice reads, copying the symbols down.

After some time, the creatures leave the small room and the bindings go slack at the same time his nasal pads flare. It is painful to sit up, but he must. Cold iron bars run on all sides. Electricity buzzes along the bars and below the surface of the floor. He turns and paces his cell. He has to know how strong the power is. If he can break out. He reaches a hand forward.

He cannot escape.

A creature comes to his cell. Strange garbled sounds issue from the being's mouth.

He realizes it is trying to talk in his language.

"Greet…Help I. Travel they." It is perplexing. The man's voice is not strong enough to make their sounds. The strange creature mews out the words and slips back into his own language. "Uh, they'll take you back to your home, but you need to make atonements first for what you stole."

The old one walks past the doorway, indifferent to his surroundings.

The captive charges the bars and nimbly slides his arm through. He pushes the creature out of the way with one arm. For beings with such power, they are light.

"Come, come, come you," he calls after the one of his own kind. The old one does not come.

There is shouting and a gigantic zap and he is down on the ground. Dazed, he is eye to eye with the body of the man who tried to speak his language. Red blood spills out of the man like a wet pouch. The smell is odd and he grows uneasy.

He only pushed the creature. It was as if the creature did not have any armor, as if he were a bag filled with soft gel and mush. His mind freezes as he realizes what he has done. He is captive but…to kill? To kill is to call for war.

He is left in the cell for days without food.

It is quiet until what he thinks is a female of the species comes in. She yells her words at him and shocks him over and over until he falls to the floor and his bowels leak out. Others come and force the female away while she makes wet noises with her nose and mouth and looks like she is in pain when she is the one hurting him.

Later, the door opens and he tenses. He is not sure if he has seen this creature before. There is no way for him to see which one is which. None of them have patterned platelets. There are no worn bristles to indicate age. He cannot read the shape of individual nasal pads. The chattering voices all sound the same and when there's more than one in a room, he has difficulty telling which one is talking.

The person says, "Greet," in his way, and continues with her strange sounds. "I know you don't understand, but I'm obligated to try. You are being charged with multiple crimes. You led your people in theft of our supplies. You should have agreed to the retribution. Instead, you purposefully killed one of our people. Someone with a family, might I add. You will be transported to Earth for a trial."

She sighs and draws a picture of a circle with arrows pointing away from it. He does not understand what those could be. He knows some markings, maps and symbols carved into certain items. He does them on specialty tools. But what the scratches on the fiber represent, he has no idea.

"Leave," she says as slowly, clearly, and loudly as she can in his language. She gestures all around her, pointing up in the air and looking upward.

He is completely bewildered by the display. Is there no war? He wonders where the old one is but is eager to leave. Longing to go home and see his partner. If she is alive, the kits will be along soon.

It feels like he lives his entire life in the cell. The creatures called humans come rarely. Then, one day, he is loaded into a vehicle. He has heard the roar and crunch of driving outside the building most days. He has anticipated leaving. It is easier this time, knowing what to expect. He will hear the burst of sound that fades to a hum and they will move. Perhaps to one of the twin cities. It has been so long, he hardly dares to hope for his hamlet. The kits will have arrived. He will have missed their first climb.

They drive a short distance and unload him. He spies a strange object, much bigger than the vehicle. It is gray and hard looking and he gets a strange sensation on his nasal pads, something he has never felt before. He senses the ache of metals but little of the dull pleasure of rock. There are sour gases like those found in the deepest of caverns and the light scent of sweat and anxiety. Humans swarm the large vehicle performing duties with urgency, but the ones at his side are resolute and determined in their pace. He does not look for long because they make him walk up a ramp, inside. He does not like this, but he cannot stop or they will shock him. They put him in a small, cramped room with his arms and feet bound. Additional restraints are added. He hollers and pleads, but they leave him. He sits for a long time until everything around him roars and shakes and he wonders why he has not yet died.

He spends a long time in the vehicle. Longer than days, longer than the great rains last. He knows they travel and move in the way of their people, but he has no idea how anything could be so far away.

They could have reached either of the twin cities many times. Where else is there to go?

Often the gibbering animals come to make their words and push limp roots through a slot. The female who attacked him before comes quietly while he is sleeping. She dips a sharp stick in his slops bucket and punctures a vulnerable spot under his leg platelet. He opens his eyes, but she is already at the door. He pours his small ration of water over the wound, then ignores it, and then scratches at it, unable to do anything else. Within one sleep, it is tender to touch. It is a weak but effective attack. He needs the pale yellow moss that grows in the caves, strong with antibacterial properties.

He tries with the one that brings food. She has never hit him before.

"Clean. Clean me."

She wrinkles the little appendage on her face when she hears his words and puts her hands in the air in a strange way. She stares at him, trying to discern his meaning but eventually leaves.

He feels hot all over, not just in his leg, though the limb pulses in a hideous way.

The next day, two of the humans enter the room and busy themselves with one of the walls. They remove a layer of the wall and pull out thin cables in several different colors.

He watches from inside the bars and decides to try it.

"No." He says their word the way they do. He does not know what it means, but he says it with that sickly nasal noise anyway. He has been practicing.

Both the animals look shocked. He gestures at his leg. "No."

The man looks at the woman. "I thought this Linkos was from the rural area. No one said it knew how to talk."

He does not know what they say, but, at last, they look at him like something other than the way he would look at a deformed sand creature. He seizes this. "No, no," he says and points to the sore area on his leg.

"Do you smell that?" the male asks.

"Since I walked in."

"No, not his smell. There's something about him that smells sick.

An infection maybe? I'll go get Dr. Jo."

Soon, a new one makes notes while talking. "D-68 is infected in the leg. The Linkos have such poor hygiene. I'm surprised it didn't happen sooner, poor thing. They're not used to being in confined quarters." She pauses while she writes on her tablet. "Bring him to the lab. Antibiotics in his food won't be enough at this point, unfortunately."

"Can't you treat it from this side of the bars, Doc?"

"I need too many supplies. Besides, if I performed the procedure here, it could get further infected."

He is dizzy and hot. He barely cares when they shackle his arms through the bars and fix a metal mesh over his mouth. He feels the weapon at his back as he stumbles along, outside the cell for the first time. He grows tired from moving his body a short way. He is supposed to be strong.

This is not strong.

They direct him from room to room until they reach a large one with a black circle in one wall. He narrows his attention on it, though he is sick. He senses that this is important. The circle is not completely black. It looks remarkably like the sky above at night, but the stars are different. They are at a new angle. It is not above him. He is...he is...in it.

He howls with rage and anger and fear and despair. How could he be in the sky, in the deep recesses of all that he pondered from his place in the hamlet long ago? He does not feel his leg or hear the humans around him. In a confused, desperate attempt, he runs headlong toward the black circle, the last thing he recognizes but does not recognize from his world.

Zaps and shocks bring him to the floor and he closes his eyes and hopes for the closure of death.

D-68 is awake, but he has been captured against a ledge for a long time. One of the things they sleep on. Everything aches and he cannot move. A human comes and dribbles water through the mesh. The water pools uncomfortably around his neck platelets, but he drinks eagerly what he can capture.

A string moves more water into his arm, tied under a small platelet, no, inserted into his very body. It is almost too much. It is cold and he can sense the liquid building up in his limb. He does not know how the water can go into an arm. Is not the mouth for drinking with these creatures?

That one comes in. The doctor looks at the monitors, records things, and looks inside D-68's eyes. Another with her, male or female, D-68 cannot tell, pushes a button that lifts his head without having to move any muscles. He feels sick with the motion.

"Well, D-68, the good news is we contained the infection and were able to keep a good portion. The bad news is the ship is going to boost soon. You're going to be safe. Uh, *safe*, where you are. Nevertheless, there might be some discomfort. Sit tight."

Now D-68 can see his feet. His legs. His leg is small. They took one of his leg platelets off. An orange-crusted white bandage wraps the limp part.

He bellows quietly, but there is not enough in him to thrash or fight. He is supposed to be strong. He must be with his kits to show them the ways. Instead, he is weak and they are taking his armor. They are taking parts of him off, and yet he is alive. He wonders how he can be who he is without himself.

The ship jumps with a jolt and he knows he is moving faster than a sand tornado, farther and farther away from his hamlet.

# Chapter 7

Yaniqui
Agriculture Planet No. 4,278

Bile burned in Yaniqui's throat. She swallowed the sour mass in time before she threw up. More than simple sickness, she felt like she'd gone from the youth of her life to a late-aged body. Yaniqui knew pain intimately, but as a self-healing humanoid, she'd never known before what it was like to fear for your own health. Now, everything was tired. Everything within her was breaking down.

    The woman that lay before Yaniqui shook her head in lingering pain. Age spots freckled her temples, creased in discomfort.

    A wow-wow-wow of whooshing emptiness swept through Yaniqui's mind. She fought to refocus as darkness crept in at the corners of her eyes. Thirst and hunger struck her as she was about to be sick, all at the same time. She took a deep breath of the iodine-scented air to remind herself where she was and what she was doing. When it was possible to refocus her eyes on the ill woman before her, she saw a thin sheet of sweat on the granny's brow.

    The old man who accompanied the woman to the infirmary prodded Yaniqui's shoulder. She realized her hands had slipped off the naked, wrinkled abdomen.

"Just a second." Yaniqui's own voice felt far away. "I need a second. I'll help you, I just—" Yaniqui stopped speaking and was dazed for a moment before the man shook her shoulder again.

"Healer, my wife is still sick. We *both* need to be in the fields in the morning or they will dock our pay."

Yaniqui felt Maemi's presence at her side. She wanted her mother to save her from this but also to never look at her mother again. Maemi was so angry. Angry that Yaniqui had shared their secret with Sario and, strangely even worse, that Yaniqui had been practicing her healing on others.

"So, it was only a matter of time until you exposed us!" Maemi had shouted in front of everyone at last meal four days ago.

No one in camp could resist a good old-fashioned family drama. Lots of people, Zimetta included, had come to Yaniqui's defense. "Nica, what would you have her do? Let people lie in pain when she could take it all away?"

Maemi turned on Zimetta like a cornered animal in possession of the finest of pelts. She put up one finger as if she could not bear to hear another inane sentence from the woman. "Zimetta, you think this is the end? We have no planet, no government. We are driftless, defenseless."

Zimetta shook her head. "As are all of us."

"No, it's different. Our gifts…make others want to take us, own us, use us for their purposes."

"I remember hearing about Wea Saa," Roh spoke up. "A whole planet of people in perfect health that could heal others. They wouldn't even let the Joint Council set up a medical station in their atmosphere." He spoke gently, "Yaniqui is an adult. Let the sick come, be healed."

"None of you understand, *none of you understand.*" Maemi cried before collapsing in the dirt. The other laborers drifted away, but that wasn't the end.

The next day, Maemi and Yaniqui worked silently in the fields. A teenager asked Yaniqui to heal his blisters at the end of the day. Mother and daughter ate and went to sleep in silence. Yaniqui didn't see Sario.

The day after, Fra Yu came. He told them they were both being transferred to the medical unit. They were to work and sleep there until further notice. Oh, and Yaniqui's leave for school was revoked.

They hadn't left since.

Maemi put a gentle hand on the man's shoulder. "Sir, my daughter is tired. She has never healed so many at a time."

"My wife is in pain."

"So is my daughter."

Yaniqui broke in. She was the one who had created all of this mess. "I just need to refresh myself for a few minutes."

The corporation doctor finally came over. Her hair hung limply in the humid heat so she was sympathetic to Yaniqui's exhaustion, if not entirely understanding. "Let the girl recover herself, Fra. She's worked hard today."

That was all Yaniqui needed. Just as a laborer couldn't leave her work unattended in the fields, Yaniqui couldn't leave her new post without permission. Yaniqui stood and made her way to the pitcher of water. Maemi sulked off in the other direction, not that Yaniqui was going to try to engage her in conversation.

The water was impossibly delicious. She drank greedily and was rewarded with a small burst of energy. Yaniqui found the bowl of food she'd set aside earlier that evening, but found her appetite didn't extend to food.

Instead, she left the stuffy room. The air outside was tepid now that the sun was down. Yaniqui's whole body tingled. It was worse than the first few days of task changes in the field—when the body went from planting to weeding or from harvesting to packing and was suddenly taken aback by the new postures and different muscle groups needed. Yaniqui's legs and shoulders weren't simply tired from bending and scooping. She was tired to her core. She pushed back her thick curls, damp at the roots with sweat. At least the sweat down her chest had dried with the cool air and, for the first time all day, things were tolerable. The single benefit to their secret being exposed was Yaniqui no longer had to wear the traditional Parentheite waist wrap.

She rubbed her hands sharply to let the burn of friction invigorate her enough to go and relieve herself at a pit. She took the long way back to the medical unit and stood outside the light of the door and windows. She stretched her neck and looked at the sky. Out there, past the moon, was a whole life she'd never have. Her chance to find Hloban was gone.

Yaniqui entered to find Maemi had healed the old woman herself. She looked as unsteady as Yaniqui and a bit of gray crossed her high cheeks. With a nod the doctor gave the mother and daughter permission to go to sleep.

Back outside, they skirted the infirmary building until they came to the door that led to their private quarters. Yaniqui was certain their new sleeping area had recently served as a broom closet. It was as bad as any cage and its location kept them on call to heal any time of the day or night.

"Psst."

Yaniqui lurched around to see a familiar face peeking out of the nearby crops. She looked at Maemi, panicked.

Maemi only waved her hand in weariness. "You'll have to talk to him at some point." She went inside without another word.

Yaniqui had been waiting years for Maemi to treat her like the woman she was. It turned out that sheer exhaustion and existential dread was all it took.

With a sigh, Yaniqui approached the wiry stalks and followed Sario in. She almost wished Maemi had forbidden her to go. It would be easier not to talk. Let him slip into the background of her life, a figure who irrevocably changed everything about her life but would go on to live his own in relative peace. They stopped in a pocket clearing between two rows.

Sario took her hands in his. His skin felt cool in the night heat. "Yaniqui, are you okay? They said you're being moved here permanently." She didn't respond so Sario took a step closer. He ran a hand up her forearm.

Yaniqui removed her hands and folded her arms. "Just for a few days longer. They're going to move us to the northern hemisphere to heal sick workers there. Or, you know, heal them there for as long as they want us to and then move us somewhere else because we have no choice." She heard Maemi's words fall from her mouth.

Sario closed nearly every gap between their bodies. "Let's go. Let's run away."

Yaniqui almost laughed to cover the threat of tears. "Run away where? This whole planet is one giant labor camp."

"We could slip onto one of the distribution vessels. You could heal someone as a bribe for a ride off. I'm sure there's someone with a sick kid."

She wanted to roll her eyes. Wanted to press her thumbs into *his* eyes. "Why would they do that when I'll already be healing their kid soon enough and then be around to heal their entire family for the rest of my life?" Yaniqui blinked back tears. "Even if I thought that would work...I wouldn't go with you."

She heard a sudden intake of breath in the darkness, but his shock only served to harden her feelings. He had to have seen this coming. There was no possible way he thought everything would go back to normal.

"You apparently don't get this yet, but we're not friends anymore. I trusted you with my family's greatest secret and you couldn't even keep it to yourself for a few days. Now Maemi is being drained half to death trying to care for so many people—"

"—I didn't realize this would happen. I mentioned your abilities to my uncle only because he was bothered by the ache in his knees. I've tried to get him switched to distribution with me, but he's still in the fields and the pain makes it hard to work." He ran a hand across his beard. "You could help a few people who need aid, that's not so terrible." He was reasoning with her. Trying to make her see it wasn't so bad after all.

It was time.

"Sario," she said, her words as hard as rock and as dirty as telefungo paste, "you should be apologizing. *Begging* me for forgiveness for ruining my life. But you're not, so let me make this abundantly clear—we have no future. And you know what? We never did."

There was blank silence among the still leaves, but Yaniqui could feel the tension of anger radiating off each of them, mingling in the night air. The two friends had always been that way. Two hot, stubborn tempers. But it was over.

"I thought you were better than this, Yaniqui. Smarter than this. Tell the corporation what you want and make a deal—you're throwing away a huge opportunity."

She knew from the break in his voice that it wasn't the opportunity she was throwing away that he cared about.

"Sario," she softened her voice. "I love someone else. I don't know how, but I'm going to get off this crisping planet and go find him." She cleared her throat. "I'm exhausted and that's all I have to say. You need to go now."

She felt more than saw him shake his head. "So, it's true. You're as obsessed with fate as they say Wea Saavians are. Everyone at camp has been talking about your weird culture. Their belief that their lives were decided when they were born. How awful it is your planet didn't help others when they had the chance. And they all died, didn't they? Now, you're going to throw away what's right in front of you for a delusion that will never come true?"

Heat rose in Yaniqui's cheeks. Hloban wasn't a delusion. "This is finished. You need to go now."

"Yeah, I see what fate brought you."

Sario pushed the plant stalks aside angrily and was gone in moments among the brush. Hot tears tracked down Yaniqui's face and an ugly snarl escaped her mouth. She wanted to stamp her feet in the dirt, chase him, hit him. Most of all, she wanted to hit herself. She was worthless. This *was* what fate brought her. A life of servitude and resentment.

"Wow, that escalated quickly."

Yaniqui whipped around to locate the husky voice. Yaniqui couldn't place it as any medical worker or laborer she had met over the past few days.

There! She spied the shadow of a figure much taller than she was. Thicker through the waist, with a pack secured to her back. Yaniqui couldn't make out the person's features, but the voice was one of power.

"Excuse me," Yaniqui said, "that was a private conversation."

"It's hard for something to be private when you're shouting it."

Yaniqui mumbled a clever "whatever" and turned to go.

"Yaniqui?"

She couldn't help but instinctively look back.

"I'll take you off this planet if you want." There was a grin in the woman's voice.

Yaniqui squinted, trying to make out her face. "Who are you?"

"Matts. I'm a bounty hunter."

Before Yaniqui could stagger a single step, the woman's hand shot out faster than a robotic arm and grasped Yaniqui by the elbow. In one twist, the woman overpowered Yaniqui and gripped her to her chest, one hand over Yaniqui's mouth, the other snapped viselike across her torso.

"I know, I know," Matts crooned. "No one likes a bounty hunter."

Yaniqui's eyes widened. The woman was off her tracks. Yaniqui struggled, but went nowhere.

Matts shushed her, kindly. "You want to get off-planet, right? Well, I'm your ticket off. I have a spacecraft. It even has seat belts. It's not the tin can most of you ride in when you come here." Matts took a deep, luxuriant breath. "Nothing beats the stink of a labor camp. This whole planet's got only a few generations before it's a dead rock. You don't want to spend your life here, Yaniqui. Your mom's invited too, of course."

Incredibly, Matts lifted her hand from Yaniqui's mouth and spun her around again. Wide leaves scratched at Yaniqui's arms.

"I know what you're thinking and, no, you're not going to scream. You're going to consider my offer. After all, you Wea Saavians have so much belief and imagination."

"How do you know about Wea Saavians?" It was the only question Yaniqui could get out.

"Oh, you're not the first one I've worked with."

For fear of turning on the lights in their bedroom and being spotted by security, Maemi lit a match and held it close to the bounty hunter's face. The slight light revealed a hatchet face with amused eyes. The hunter raised a brow, sensing Maemi's and Yaniqui's assessment.

"She said she could take us off-planet," Yaniqui started.

"They," Matts corrected. "And I can. Isn't that what both of you want most?"

Maemi dropped the match in shock. "Yaniqui," her voice warned, "they are not going to helpfully take us off-planet and let us go—they're going to kidnap us, sell us, and—"

"And your life will be a lot better than it is now," they said.

Maemi reached for Yaniqui and clutched her to her side.

"Let's do this the easy way," Matts said. "You're thinking about screaming. I'll be gone before the guards get here. Then I'll sneak in another night, sedate you, and take you away. So, let's be clear—I'm not giving you a choice of whether you're leaving this planet with me. I'm giving you the choice of *how*. It's an important distinction."

Maemi muttered to herself and pushed her curls out of her face. "My daughter and I are not going with you."

Matts's smile was easy to see because their teeth glinted in the moonlight.

"You're lucky to have the opportunity. When the news of two Wea Saavians' sudden appearance on an random ag. planet came through the channels, you can be sure there was an uproar. I'm lucky I was already on-planet for…some other work. Others, well, they'll be here by tomorrow afternoon at the latest and I'll have trouble keeping them off you if we're still here."

Maemi hung her head. "News of us is on the Interstellar Wave?"

Matts shook their head. "Not yet. Only on less clean channels. But Akar knows and put a bounty on your two lovely heads, and these days that's just as, if not more, powerful than the public discourse."

"Akar." Maemi didn't pose the word as a question but in disbelief.

"That's who you'd sell us to?" Yaniqui asked.

"Listen, kid, I know it's not what you wanted to do when you woke up this morning, but that boy was right. You can't control everything—and fate definitely isn't going to do that for you. But you can decide some things. You have bargaining power. Cooperation goes a long way with companies like these. Let them buy you from me and sell you to some wealthy family in Selruit. You'll be taken care of and you'll service a lot fewer people than you are here. Wealthy families know about maintaining property."

Chills went down Yaniqui's back. This was becoming more real by the minute. She was not just a debt-ridden, indentured laborer. She was going to be owned, a real slave.

There was the sound of a machine and a shout. Yaniqui knew what a late-night arrival meant. Someone was hurt and a staff member would fetch them shortly. Maemi waved her hands frantically in front of her face as if to dispel the bounty hunter.

Heavy footsteps crunched outside and their door unceremoniously flew open. Yaniqui looked around in terror, but Matts was gone, as if by magic.

The nurse stuck her head in. "*I said*," said the nurse, "there's more patients." She gave Maemi the once-over. "Put your pants back on and *come on*."

Before the door swung shut, Yaniqui and Maemi made eye contact. The ascending moonlight illuminated exhausted terror on both their faces.

Matts's voice came from the darkness. "Well?"

# Chapter 8

Hloban
New Washington, WI, Earth

Loera was helping Obani put unlit sparklers on the indigo cake and Hloban was hanging color-changing balloons when the kitchen wall ticker glowed. An urgent ring boomed through the house. It was a call from Emmett.

Hloban hadn't expected to hear from Secretary-General Cortez's office again so soon. Perhaps they wanted to schedule a debrief.

"Sorry, I had no idea they were going to call. If you need help, I can pretend I didn't hear it—"

Loera waved him off. "Oh yes," Loera said, "please miss your call with the United Nations. I just simply cannot handle the balloons by myself."

Hloban would have thought of something funny to say back, but he was already darting up the stairs to his office, his mind racing as he tried to figure out what they could possibly want on the weekend. Once inside, door shut, he pushed a button.

"Hello, this is Hloban speaking."

"Please hold for the secretary-general."

"What? Fuck, Emmett. What's this about?" Hloban made to grab his supplies to take notes, but he tripped over a set of toy buildables Obani had dragged in the day before.

He'd never been connected directly to Cortez before. He was a consultant on interstellar diplomatic matters. All of his projects started slowly months in advance and culminated with long, boring meetings. What awful sequence of events had happened to spark this impromptu call?

"Mr. Milson, I have some news for you."

"Madam Secretary-General," Hloban stammered. He kicked the toys out of the way and lunged for his notebook. "How can I help you?"

"My office received a report from the Joint Council a short while ago. It seems a Wea Saavian, Yaniqui Daful, has been found and is currently in the possession of Akar Enterprises."

Every word out of the United Nations secretary-general's mouth shocked Hloban more deeply than the last until the Earth fell away completely. His head went fuzzy and he reached his chair just in time to drop in heavily.

"Emmett," Cortez demanded. "Did we lose the blasted signal again? I don't understand why of all the phones on the planet—"

Her voice broke through his fog of disbelief. Hloban bolted upright out of his chair as if he was a naughty child found playing with his dad's work things. "I'm here, Madam Secretary-General. I apologize. I thought you said…a Wea Saavian has been found."

"Yes, a young woman."

Hloban's hands shook. They were shaking and they couldn't stop. It suddenly occurred to Hloban to wonder why the secretary-general herself was calling with the news. He swallowed, trying to consider how to ask just that when she answered the question for him.

"You're going to go get her for us."

When Hloban finally made his way downstairs, he opened his mouth to speak to his wife and try to find some words to describe the unbelievable and fraught news he had just gotten.

A knock at the door came first. Obani ran whooping and

screaming to let in a friend from school and her parents. A few more people trickled in and then, like a ship's ignition, they flooded. Loera's family and Obani's playdate buddies and respective parents and other expats piled winter jackets and boots in the foyer until they made a small mountain.

Hloban hovered at Loera's elbow, but she was entrenched in a conversation with Steph's mom who would return in an hour but had brought a container of approved snacks. Couldn't the lady see he needed to talk to his wife? He had to unburden himself with what Cortez had just put on him.

"*Irizolz ku*, Obani."

Hloban twisted around to see his kinsman Keyad wish Obani a happy birthday.

Hloban didn't care who took in his wild eyes and gaping mouth. He was just realizing how messy things were about to get.

Obani.

Hloban had chosen Obani's name. He had explained to Loera that in Wea Saavian culture there was a process to creating the name based on the partners' names. He didn't elaborate on exactly how, but he once overheard Loera telling her mother that the *O* was shared in both of their names, so it actually made a lot of sense.

It was true, he had created the true name of his son. But he did not use Loera's name. He used Yaniqui's. In memorial.

Now, watching his son gleefully receive a present to put in his gift pile, Hloban wondered at the wisdom of the choice he had made four years ago. As a Wea Saavian, Keyad had likely already figured it out, but he wasn't one to jar the cruiser. Hloban's heart sped at the thought of having that conversation with Loera.

Hloban walked back to the kitchen with the intention of pretending to be a good host until he could pull Loera upstairs and tell her what happened. He put strips of masking tape on cups and wrote kids' names on them so they could keep some semblance of personal boundaries alive at the preschooler-infested event.

"Hloban."

He jumped, spilling the empty cups all over the counter.

Amanda, Keyad's wife, looked at him in surprise. Then she

laughed. "I just wanted to say I'm putting this dish in the oven to keep warm."

"Oh, it's fine, it's fine…" he trailed off as he stood the cups upright. He was starting to get the sense that he wasn't fine.

A herd of kids ran shrieking through the kitchen followed closely behind by another with some gods-awful roaring dinosaur toy. Hloban had nearly finished writing names on cups when the kids ran through again and one ran full-tilt into his legs. Hloban knocked half the cups down again.

Hloban wanted peace and quiet to consider all Cortez had said. Instead, his house was full of people.

Hloban found himself in the living room next to Keyad who handed him a wrapped gift. Hloban tucked it clumsily under his arm, not caring what was inside.

"I don't think I had half this many friends when I was Obani's age," Keyad said.

Hloban smiled weakly but couldn't think of a response. Adam appeared at his dad's side with a drink, still in his winter jacket.

He should say something. Hloban had to force his brain to think.

"Adam, I didn't expect to see you today," he finally came up with. He would have supposed a fresh college grad would have better things to do. Though actually, Adam wasn't a recent graduate anymore. Watching Adam grow up over the past several years and now having Obani made Hloban group himself with Keyad. Plus, they were the only individuals on-planet with any memories of Wea Saa. It looked like that was about to change. Hloban put his hands in his pockets to stop them from shaking.

Adam pushed his parka hood back revealing shaggy black hair. It was clear the three men with dark hair and bronzed skin were family of some kind. "I came home for the weekend." He looked around to see who was closest to them. "Actually, I had to visit the *conscru*." Hloban's ears pricked. It was the nickname he and Keyad gave to any government office. It meant *irksome nuisance* on Wea Saa. "There was a problem with an application."

Hloban was instantly on the alert. As a half-Wea Saavian, anything that affected Adam could someday do the same to Obani.

"I applied to work at a mining company in the Haemea Star System."

Hloban shot a look at Keyad and decided Keyad was dismayed by the choice of company too. "You don't want to work for a mining company, do you?"

Adam slid his coat off and hung it over a couch arm. "I'd work for any company in space at this point. But my application's being withheld. Immigration Services doesn't want to give me permission to work off-planet." Though eager to share his disgust at his current predicament, Adam paused to shove a handful of chips into his mouth.

A boisterous laugh came from the kitchen and Hloban knew instantly that Jeb had arrived. It was more than a bit alarming when the large, shaggy animoid laughed. "Jeb" was a culturally offensive nickname that Jeb didn't mind. His real name sounded to Hloban generally like growly noises. He was a good three feet taller than Hloban and had to duck through the doorways. Loera wasn't entirely sure having Jeb at a children's birthday party was appropriate, but Hloban had only shrugged. Jeb was one of the few friends he had that was not Loera's friend first.

The only person Hloban expected to arrive, and hadn't, was Waquas, but Jeb was much more comfortable making Earthlings and humanoids uncomfortable than Waquas was. With his size, brown hairy body, and big personality, it was practically a daily to-do list item for Jeb.

The aforementioned Steph was caught with a bag of chocolate chips just as one of the other preschool parents spilled a bottle of beer on the couch. With a smile, Hloban assured him it was fine though it pissed him off. *He* wouldn't have put out fermented drinks at a child's birthday, but it was Wisconsin.

He took the cushion back to the laundry room, pleased for an excuse to be alone. The conversation with Cortez ran circles in his head.

"I beg your pardon," Hloban had stuttered. He genuinely hadn't understood the sequence of words that had come out of Cortez's mouth.

"I said you're going to go get the woman."

"Yaniqui?"

"Yes, Mr. Milson, I'm sure this is a shock, but this is great news for her, for you, and for Earth. You're going to retrieve her and bring her back." Cortez was positively jovial. She likely didn't get to give good news often in her job, and here she was, telling a member of an endangered race that another member had been found.

Hloban took a shallow breath and wondered if he was going to pass out. "Madam Secretary-General. I was betrothed. Engaged. To this girl. Woman." Oh gods, he was oversharing. He licked his lips. "And now I am married."

There was an uncomfortable pause and Hloban could hear someone snicker in Cortez's office. Probably Emmett, that traitor.

"Yes, well," Cortez said brandishly, "it sounds like there's some, ah, details to be figured out, but Emmett is going to make arrangements for your departure."

"Departure? You can't be serious." Hloban realized he was being too familiar with the most powerful woman in the solar system. "What I mean is, I can't just leave Earth."

"Immigration won't be very happy with me," Cortez conceded, "but I'm sure we can push through the red tape and carry on. One of our pilots will take you out there and bring the Wea Saavian here. To Earth."

Shit. Deyo and Kilberg were right. Cortez didn't want to wait generations to make Earth a voting member on the Joint Council. She wanted to stack things in her favor now. How perfect would it be for Cortez to continue providing a home to every known Wea Saavian in the galaxy? Keyad had been on Earth before Wea Saa was destroyed. Then Hloban came. They both had sons. That was great and all, but a Wea Saavian woman? That would put Earth on the map.

Cortez was still talking. Hloban couldn't help but interrupt.

"I really can't go. My family—"

"Now, Mr. Milson, before you start giving me all of that, rest assured, we'll pay your consulting fee for your work on this project. Please understand it's very important to Earth that this woman be brought to safety and live here."

"Again, I can't just leave and go on a rescue mission to save the last Wea Saavian..." he trailed off, because why the hell not? Why couldn't he go and save one of his people who was scared and alone? And the fact that they had been betrothed a long time ago...Hloban pushed that nugget to the back of his mind to dwell on what that might mean later.

"Mr. Milson, you've applied through various offices for information on any possible survivors of Wea Saa. When you first arrived on Earth, you put in a missing person's report for this woman's exact case number. It seems as if you've been searching for others of your kind for years, even specifically for this woman." She spoke in that voice she got when she knew she was being persuasive. "It would seem like the person on Earth with the most knowledge of the Joint Council would be the exact right person to save this Wea Saavian."

She was flattering him—Jeb was the most knowledgeable being on Earth regarding the Joint Council—but in an instant, he knew he was going to do what Cortez demanded of him. Go and get Yaniqui. Celebrate that she was alive. Bring her to Earth.

He ran a hand through his short hair. Really? Just like that?

"If I'm going, I'm piloting my ship with a crew of my choosing."

A voice came on that Hloban couldn't place—probably someone to keep Cortez from having to argue with a bewildered alien. "Mr. Milson, one of our ships will do the job well. It will be most advantageous—"

"Do you have a plan for how to get her? You're not planning on *buying* Yaniqui from Akar, are you?"

"Of course not—"

"If I'm going, I'm taking my craft. I'm not getting stuck between star systems because someone else misread a gauge before takeoff."

"That wouldn't happen—" the nameless voice on the call started.

Cortez popped on. "Fine." He could almost hear her wave a hand in dismissal. "But you're taking our crew members. And that's not up for debate. You need clearance to leave and you'll only get that clearance if we have Earth crew members on board with you for the rescue mission."

There hadn't been time to argue and Hloban hadn't had the wits to do so.

"Hoban," Loera called to the laundry room. "Let's do the cake."

Hloban stared at the cushion he was supposed to be cleaning. The beer stain had turned into a huge water stain, but he would deal with it later.

He left the laundry room and everyone gathered around the kitchen table. Obani bounced in his seat and smiled big when his mom picked up the indigo layer cake and brought it over. Four sparkling candles reflected in Loera's glasses as she set it in front of Obani.

A sudden *ding* rang over the not-visible-but-not-invisible speakers. Another alert, but—damn it.

Hloban forgot to disconnect the Wave. The notice scrolling on the wall ticker was not from a local source but from an interstellar news bureau. The device had been plugged in since the previous day. How much was that going to cost him?

Loera set the cake down. "What? How are we getting an off-planet notice?"

Everyone looked up and read the text—Personal alert: Wea Saavian female, declared.

It went quiet. Hloban's heart stopped too quickly to notice Keyad exchange a look with Amanda or see Loera cover her mouth.

"Do my birthday song," Obani said. "I would like four songs because I am four."

Hloban made eye contact with Loera and gave a desperate, silent plea as he stumbled away from the crowd. If this news was public, there was no way he would not be the first one to know what the hell was going on. In the hall, Loera's dad grabbed his arm to steady him and he wrenched it away. Hloban went to his office and lurched over his chair as he made his way to the wall screen. It wasn't only that news outlet. There were other headlines.

*Declared endangered species located.*

*Self-healing medical research gets a boon.*

What was the impetus to Yaniqui's discovery? Had she been with Akar this whole time and they were just now leaking the information? Otherwise, if Yaniqui had been alive, wouldn't he have found mention of her over the years? Or wouldn't she have found him? Had he made himself too hard to locate, trying to protect himself and later Obani, as well as Keyad and Adam? Had she even been looking for him?

From downstairs, he heard the rush of whispers grow to a boom of conversation. Jeb's baritone voice rumbled.

Hloban took a series of fast shallow breaths. He didn't want to hear any of it. He was suddenly sure his ears were going to pop. He sat down. The thoughts came quickly. Yani was really alive. At the root of it, none of the questions mattered. It was time to move. He rushed to his bedroom and threw clothes and official markers and stuff in a bag.

"Hoban?"

Hloban turned and saw his wife in the doorway.

"Loera, I have to go and help this Wea Saavian."

Loera looked at the bag closely. "Go get her? Like a rescue?"

"That was the call I took before the party started. Cortez asked me to go."

"Hoban, you're a consultant. You're hardly qualified—"

"It's Yaniqui."

There was never such a still quiet as when Loera stopped talking.

"Yanakey...the girl you were arranged to marry? But she's dead."

"Apparently not. I don't know if she was in hiding or if Akar had her this whole time, but I need to go now. I need to talk to her."

"But, Hoban, you can't leave. Your business. And the birthday party. You don't know where she is or how long it will take. If you need to talk to her, just make a fucking phone call," she shrieked the last sentence.

The buzz of conversation downstairs faltered.

Hloban led Loera to the bed and sat her down in a patch of afternoon light stretched across the blankets. "I know. I was stunned too. But she's out there. I have to go get her."

"Why, Hoban? Why you?"

"Who else would? Loera, our families were bound to each other. I have a responsibility to her. She's completely alone, scared out of her mind, I'm sure. Akar's going to—"

"Okay, okay. I just can't believe this little girl has been out there this whole time. She must be terrified. To go through all that as a kid."

As Loera took a sharp breath through her nose and composed

herself, Hloban realized there was something else he had done years ago that he regretted. Long ago, when they were talking about getting married, Hloban had told Loera he had been engaged before. He told her everything he could about the betrothal, partly to set the woman he loved at ease, and partly because he was still mourning the woman he had expected to love. It had been a long time since he talked with someone about Yaniqui.

In the conversation, Loera seemed to take great solace in the fact that Hloban said Yaniqui had been much younger than him. And maybe he didn't so much as mistakenly leave his wife with the wrong impression but actively fostered it to make her feel better. Whenever it was brought up, he downplayed how much he cared for Yaniqui, partly because of the age gap. He didn't expect it to ever be a problem. She was *dead* and talking about stars and shit made him sound kooky.

The thing was, Yaniqui was only something like five years younger than him. It felt like a big difference when he was on Wea Saa, but when they both finished their apprenticeships and married as adults, the gap would have been nothing. Loera was actually older than Hloban was, but she had been happy to go on believing Hloban had never been in love with anyone else, never thought of the life he was supposed to have all because it was an arrangement between two people of slightly different ages.

*Fuck.*

"Loera, I'm sorry," he said, not totally sure what his apology encapsulated. "I'm sorry it's so fast. Cortez says I need to get to her before she disappears again." He pressed harder. He needed to make her understand. "She's the last family I have left. She might be the only other Wea Saavian out there. And she's my responsibility."

Loera swallowed. Hloban saw the shock leave her face and her normal control filter in.

"I don't understand, but you're right, if you can help this kid...just don't get yourself captured. Make Cortez give you diplomatic immunity or something."

It was all becoming very real very fast. Hloban was close to shaking. He'd thought if he ever discovered another Wea Saavian, he'd feel elated, but instead he felt sick. The shock and full burden of what he was realizing was just hitting him.

Loera turned over his bag and a jumbled set of clothes and papers fell out. "I'll pack for you. Send everyone home."

Hloban was at the door when Loera called out again. "You better…"

Hloban turned.

She shook her head, close to tears, and turned back to her task. "Never mind."

Hloban's head swam with preparation lists as he went downstairs, ready to tell the party guests to go home. Everyone lifted their gazes from the floor to stare at him and he had to remind himself that most of them didn't know he had any personal connection to the news story. He didn't exactly go around the capital telling parents at dance class that he was one of the last of his race.

Jeb had used the Wave connection to pull up a brief article on the story. Hloban stood rigid, cursing every god he could think of, which was just his own, but took the opportunity to read the full story quickly. There were few facts, and they all centered around one: Yaniqui was in custody with a slaver.

"Akar…" Keyad said slowly. They met each other's glance. It was the worst-case scenario.

Hloban took a deep breath, but it made sense. Everything from there on linked swiftly in his brain. Yaniqui was missing for a decade—since the solar flare—then was suddenly plastered across the news. Found and put up for sale. It was something he had considered before. No common surrogate or slave could do what she could do, and everyone already wanted to own one of them. Like him, Yaniqui could heal herself. But she was also gifted with the ability to heal others. All Wea Saavian women were. Her self-healing, lifesaving genes would pass on to female children and grandchildren. She was the closest thing to invincible possible. Everyone would want to use her. Medical research centers. Mercenaries. Kingpins. Business tycoons.

Human trafficking, labor internment, and outright slavery weren't unheard of. Hloban had just listened to a podcast on asteroid miners, enslaved workers held deep in space, but it was entirely different seeing the last female of Wea Saa, his female, in custody, sale pending.

Hloban looked at the group assembled in his house.

"I guess everyone knows now. It's true—I've been consulting on a big case for a human rights firm trying to locate this woman." Hloban tried to keep his face as neutral as possible. "I need to act fast if she is going to have any chance at freedom. Sorry everyone, we'll have to have you over a different time."

"But I am four," Obani said to the quiet kitchen.

# Chapter 9
Adam (*A-dam*)
New Washington, WI, Earth

Adam sat down next to Obani with a slice of birthday cake. Of those left—Adam's parents, Hloban's family, and Jeb—only Adam and Obani ate cake. With the final guests seen to the door, Hloban came back to the kitchen looking like a different person. When Adam first arrived at the party, he couldn't help but feel like a tagalong kid seeing the inside of someone's perfect life. Hloban and Loera, effortlessly sophisticated, had everything anyone could ever want. Now, Hloban's eyes were red and deadened. He moved as if in a daze, his thoughts clearly elsewhere.

Adam took a bite. It was mostly frosting. He took another bite of frosting and realized the edge of the cake didn't start where he thought it did.

Hloban wondered out loud if anyone had believed him. Adam couldn't care less if the preschool crew believed Hloban's lie about how he was involved in finding and representing the "last Wea Saavian." Representing how? Hloban was a glorified hand-holder for out-of-the-loop Earthling business leaders and government officials.

Adam's question was bigger. The answer would shape the rest of his life.

He finished the cake, real cake now, in five big bites.

The door creaked and a gust of chilled wind filtered through the house. Loera was still nowhere to be found so Adam knew it was a parent returning for a missing stuffed animal or some such thing.

"Waquas," Jeb acknowledged the newcomer with his low, raspy voice.

Waquas brought the cold air into kitchen with him. Still wearing a dark bomber jacket, his cheeks burned dark green with cold. Waquas pulled off his thick hat to reveal a bald head, the same green as the rest of his body. He rubbed his cheeks with his hands as if to warm them. He arched his hairless brows and Adam sensed the flavor of the room from Waquas's perspective: a kid's birthday as stiff and awkward as a college party broken up by seething parents.

"Well, are we going?" Waquas asked.

Adam smiled. That was exactly what he wanted to know.

Immigration blocking his off-planet applications was only the most recent occurrence to prolong Adam's unemployment. He'd had an actual job interview the day before—not an assessment test or a video call, but in person, at an office. Going in, Adam actually thought the space tourism company would hire him. But once he got there, they started interviewing him to work as an assistant in scheduling. The base pay would barely cover his student loans.

"Ah, I think there must be a miscommunication. I'm applying to be a tour manager." Taking low-atmosphere trips with rich people seemed like the first step to actually getting out there.

The woman interviewing him had smoothed her long hair down, practically petting it. Her lips formed a round O as she tapped quickly through the files. "Yes, that's right, you did."

Adam smiled.

"It looks like you were automatically downgraded for lack of space experience."

Adam leaned forward. He remembered the coaching his dad had given him. "I think I'd be an excellent tour manager."

"But you haven't been to space."

"I will if you take me there."

She looked again at her computer in confusion. "You want to book a trip?"

"No. What I mean," Adam enunciated carefully, "is I can *get* the experience. You know, on the job."

The interview ended shortly thereafter and Adam had driven to his parents' house for another long weekend of hanging out with them between interviews. But now, Adam sensed a real opportunity.

"How do you know about the found Wea Saavian?" Keyad asked Waquas.

"I saw it on the train news panel on my way here. You're going to go get her, right?" Waquas directed the last part to both Hloban and Keyad.

Everyone looked at Hloban. He gave a stiff nod.

"She's really a Wea Saavian like you?" Jeb asked. "I thought the last of your kind were here on Earth under the Protective ACT."

Adam put his plate in the dishwasher. His thoughts were no longer with the group. As a half-Wea Saavian, he always assumed Hloban, Obani, and his dad were the only other ones. It wasn't that news of the girl's survival was unimportant to Adam, but his own impending opportunity seemed much more pertinent.

Keyad answered, "That we knew of. We thought there might be others, but never expected we'd find them. Anyone still alive would be in hiding."

His mom finished the thought. "Out in the open like this is a huge risk." Lines creased around her mouth as she looked at Adam out of the corner of her eye.

Jeb growled softly. "You could apply for action from the Joint Council, but the laws surrounding this are watertight." He paused, as if steeling himself to continue. Or convincing himself someone had to say it. "If she sold herself to Akar, and you know they will claim she did and have doctored evidence even if she didn't, she's never getting out. She's going to be sold to some ultrawealthy political type or a military venture that would make good use of on-demand healing. They're going to—"

"Stop! I know." Hloban put his hands up as if he could shield himself from the rest of that statement. "I'm not applying for fucking action. I'm going. I would hope I would do the same for anyone left with our blood, but this is more than that. I knew her. Yaniqui and I were betrothed. There's no way I can leave her."

Adam knew about the hokey Wea Saavian nonsense his dad grew up with, and Hloban was still in deep. There was no way *he* was going to marry someone based on the placement of the stars and blindly expect fate to plan out his life. Adam shifted his gaze away from Hloban. His cheeks and ears begin to warm and he tried to stall the blush. He didn't want anyone making the wrong assumption that he was interested in Hloban's lost romantic life or that he himself (for gods' sake!) would be interested in the girl that way, when in fact he was blushing because he was embarrassed *for* Hloban. Adam had heard enough about betrothal and star destinies to know it was a sentimental piece of Wea Saavian culture. He wanted nothing to do with it and, as an American, it embarrassed him that his ancestors had based their lives and love around the random placement of the stars.

But if that's what Hloban believed and because of that had to leave Earth to go save someone, Adam was going too. Even if he had to stow away on the spaceship and eat half rations.

"I'm going too," Keyad said. "It's my moral responsibility."

"I'm going as well," Waquas stated simply. "I need to leave the Sol System so I can renew my visa upon reentry."

"That's not a good reason to go all that way, Waquas," Amanda said.

"No, but I'd be going anyway." Waquas sat down with a slice of cake. His slice looked more normal than Adam's misshapen one. "Happy birthday, Obani. You get bigger every time I see you."

Obani was sitting in Amanda's lap, almost asleep, and didn't respond. He was pouting and talking to no one because his party was canceled. Though a warm, empathetic lap was always welcome.

Adam wondered why Waquas would want to travel across the galaxy to save the girl—Waquas wasn't Wea Saavian. Adam wasn't actually sure what Waquas was. He had the same body build as a human but did his green marbled skin mean he wasn't a humanoid? But Adam had to seize his own moment. He cleared his throat and said as offhandedly as he could, "I think it's my moral responsibility too. We need to go get the girl."

Amanda sat up suddenly, causing Obani to whine in protest, and started talking, reasoning why Adam couldn't go.

At the same time, Hloban rolled his eyes and said, "You've never even been in space, Adam."

"Waquas, this is an extended journey. I can't imagine you're able to swing that," Keyad said.

"I'll make arrangements."

Amanda spoke gently to her son, but her words still stung. "I believe there were people in need yesterday too, but that didn't force you off-planet to go and save *them*."

"No, no, no," Hloban shouted. His skin darkened and suddenly he was pacing and storming the kitchen. He threw a dish down in the sink and it shattered.

Obani put his hands over his face and watched his father through his fingers.

"The U.N. is already insisting I take their crew members. This is big enough already. Just Waquas and I are going." Hloban stopped and closed his eyes. He opened them and waved Keyad down who had opened his mouth. "Obani, I'm sorry. Daddy's very stressed right now. I made a bad choice." He looked at the room. "I know you're trying to help," Hloban continued, fighting for control of his voice, "but I need to leave as soon as possible. Too many people will slow things down. What if Yani disappears before I can get to her?"

Keyad put both hands up before he started talking, as if negotiating with a furious Jeb instead of short-statured Hloban. "You have to let me go," Keyad said. "There's no way I'm leaving what could be the last one of us out there in danger."

Hloban hesitated, then said, "If you're sure."

Keyad nodded.

Adam leaned forward to speak, but his mother carefully handed Obani to Waquas, then bodily yanked Adam up out of his chair and pushed him into the hallway. His father followed.

"No. Absolutely not." Amanda shook her head.

Adam turned to them, prepared. "I know I don't have experience in space," he tried to use his most I'm-a-grown-up-who-doesn't-need-to-beg-you voice, "but I think it'd be best if I went with Dad and Hloban to rescue the girl."

"Adam," his mom said heatedly. "You can't go. There's too much danger. Things you've never even thought about. Do you want to risk your life for someone you've never met?"

"Dad's going."

"Well, it's Dad's moral responsibility."

"And I think I can help. Dad wasn't living on Wea Saa when it blew up. He was here. With you. If he still feels such an obligation to his people, how can I stay here while they save the girl without me?"

"What's her name?" Amanda challenged her son, less angry now than sensibly direct.

"Yankey," Adam responded confidently.

Amanda brushed back her flaxen hair and folded her arms. "That's not even it. Tell me true, Adam. Why?"

His dad stood quiet in Hloban's hallway. Adam shifted his weight. When he woke up that morning, all he wanted was for his paperwork to come off without a hitch. Now, his entire future came down to the next five minutes.

"It'd be worth it—all the last members of the race finally together, working together."

"So, bringing the survivors together is the big idea? What if the three of you are on the same ship and it explodes?" his mother asked. "Wouldn't it be better for you to stay here as collateral?"

Adam rolled his eyes. "Space travel is growing safer all the time. Besides, we took a plane to the Californian Edge, didn't we? That's statistically as dangerous as piloting ships within our solar system."

"And once you get beyond that?" His dad's shoulders hunched. "Traveling faster than light speed is the most dangerous thing I've ever done. And when we get there…we either have to find the money to purchase Yaniqui or steal her. This isn't a research trip. Adam, you don't know what life out there is like. These corporations are vicious. They're not just business entities. They have complete control over vast areas of the galaxy. The *Joint Council* goes up against them and loses. We likely will not do better."

Out of the corner of Adam's eye, he caught his mother's expression at her husband's admission and he had to steady himself to keep advocating. He *had* to go. He'd tried for the past six years to compete his way into a space program for young people, to no avail. Every internship had a line of exceptionally qualified students who also wanted to go into space, and he'd started thinking they all must be gifted in a way he was not because they were the ones asked to go.

"If I don't go now, I may never get my chance to go to space." Tears pricked at the back of Adam's eyes. It was the truest thing he said yet. "Part of my history is out there, and if I stay on Earth, I want to know it's because I chose it. Not because I was randomly born here instead of there."

His mom stared at his face so intently, Adam looked away. She looked upset, and worse than that, she was trying to control her emotions and failing. Her chin trembled. Adam knew she was steeling herself to break his heart with a *no*.

She took his hand. "Okay."

It wasn't clear who was more shocked, Adam or his father.

His mom could barely get the words out. She covered her grimace with a strange, small smile. "I know you're running out of chances. And, yes, I think you have to help that girl. But remember, Adam, even if people here look past the Earthling in you and see only the Wea Saavian, know you have the right to be here."

"And none of where we ended up is an accident," his dad said. "I don't want you to feel like you have to choose between this dangerous thing or living a life of boredom. There's a middle ground, you know."

Adam nodded and pretended to be more contemplative than he felt. "I don't believe in destiny or anything, but all of this does feel right. We'll go and help that girl and I'll finally have a step that will lead me to a career."

"That was supposed to be college."

"I guess it's going to be a family vacation."

Adam followed his parents back into Hloban's kitchen, elated. He'd finally get to do it. Experience life off Earth. He had grown up in the decades after Contact, but Earth was still behind the wider galaxy in a number of ways. It was partly his civic duty to build that bridge. It was a race to see what private investor could get out there and make connections. There was a lot of business to be done out there. Why not by him?

They returned to the kitchen, and Keyad gave Hloban a nod.

Hloban groaned slightly and turned to Jeb. "And what's your issue?" he demanded. "You have some sort of moral responsibility issue too? Or do you want to pad your resume?" He jerked his head at Adam.

"That's not what I'm doing," Adam started, though it was exactly what he was doing.

Jeb laughed a rumbling cough. "There's no way I'm going to take on a corporation like Akar to save someone I don't know." He shook his head and the long, thick fur on the sides of his face trembled. "But I'll help expedite your clearance to launch." Government officials rarely said no to Jeb, a combination of his imposing size and fear of being accused of speciesism.

Waquas turned to Keyad. "Hloban's ship is still out at my place, but we'll bring it to the Winslow Space-Earth Station for prelaunch checks."

The group broke up, talking about preparations.

Loera walked in with a small bag, her face a mask. It finally clicked with Adam. For him, this was an adventure. For Hloban and Loera, this was personal.

Adam had heard Hloban talk about Wea Saa before and the beautiful girl he was supposedly linked to by destiny as decided by the stars and yada yada yada.

Adam never heard Loera talk about her husband's home planet, but he did once hear her mention "the girl Hloban was traditionally engaged to a long time ago."

And now Hloban was crossing the galaxy to go get her.

# Chapter 10
Ippa
In Transit

Ippa slept for fourteen hours straight. She woke exhausted and dull and felt out of sorts trying to place where she was supposed to be, what she was supposed to be doing.

In a flash, the conversation in Professor Jinu's office came spilling back. Her "idiosyncratic presentation." All that Jinu implied about her lack of ability as a student. The wild thing was that Ippa had done the assignment! And crisping better than anyone else. Who else had written code to make a holograph of their planet? Who else ran simulations of Original Nine DNA to see how Earth's habitat may have changed it?

A nagging voice told Ippa it was easier for her to believe she was *overqualified* for the galaxy's preeminent university rather than not good enough, but she ignored it. As an adult no longer tied to the academic system, she could ignore those little voices now.

Ippa fumed, restless in her dorm, but she didn't dare show her face in public. She was sure word about her expulsion—her entire failure of a life—traveled quickly among the population of perfect students, always in competition for the next high marks. She allowed Bel in her room to say goodbye while she packed, the only being she saw since Professor Jinu dashed her dreams.

The amphibian told Ippa, "You'll find your place soon. You're so driven, how could you not?"

Bel's expression was hard to read as always, but Ippa thought she read disdain in it. Bel interlaced her long fingers, fidgeting.

"The Shou was supposed to be my place, Bel. I've spent my entire life working to get *here*." Even as she confessed her failures, she fought back emotion. Ippa had already decided she wasn't going to cry in front of anyone, even though her entire self-worth and life plan depended on The Shou, and she had no idea what she was going to do instead.

"Ippa, you're a college student. You're not that old."

It was all cozy-feeling sentiments and nothing else. Ippa would probably say the exact same thing if her friend had been expelled. It was okay for anyone else not to be good enough, as long as you were more than enough.

She turned to snap at Bel, but forced herself to calmly say, "Would you return these to the library? I'd rather not go back." She stacked the six books she had so recently signed out and held them out to Bel.

There was the briefest hesitation. "Sure, Ippa."

Once Bel left with the library books, Ippa realized she had dressed that morning in her Shou uniform to no end. She had fought so hard to get one but lost the battle to be comfortable in it. She took it off for the last time and folded it gently. Still in her underwear, she burrowed under her blankets again, tucked them so that her freckled nose peeked out, and went back to sleep.

She slept for only another two hours, but for the first time in a long time, Ippa almost felt rested. But not peaceful. She was even resentful of the fact that she had enjoyed the sleep, as if it meant she was too soft for The Shou.

Instead of continuing to wear her uniform, study in the biblioplaza, and spend every waking hour researching, writing, and presenting—all to build her mind, learn everything, and become a force to be reckoned with along the way—Ippa finished packing.

A day later, she boarded a small traditional cruiser that took her and two dozen others to just outside the atmosphere where they prepared to board a commercial shuttle built to maximize space and efficiency. With no artificial gravity, seats were set in stationary rings around the circumference of the shuttle body. No one giggled during the weightless boarding—with a flight full of adjunct professors and students going out on field studies, it wasn't that sort of crowd—but Ippa found she couldn't even enjoy the novelty. Once she found her seat number, a crew member strapped her in tightly. Passengers sat on either side of Ippa, in front of her, behind her, as well as above her. The empty space in the middle of the ring of seated passengers was just big enough to let a crew member glide through double-checking all the harnesses were secure.

It was nearly as full as the biblioplaza. Ippa took a deep breath. It emerged as a snort.

The craft launched smoothly and pockets of chatter sprang up throughout the vessel. Screens popped to life among the seats and Ippa's neighbor took out a liquid meal pouch.

She had plenty of time to consider her plans. The most obvious was to return home. But how could she show up at her maternal family compound, scaring them half to death as they didn't expect to see her until Level Two break, and then face their disappointment in her disgrace? Or worse, their pleasure at her return-inducing failure? Her mother would be only too happy to have Ippa back. She'd want Ippa to attend a nice, on-planet technical school and go into spacecraft manufacturing like the rest of them. Ippa couldn't handle that bland career, and her mother was at the top of the long list of things she couldn't face.

A smooth voice announced they reached Verde Outpost 9,870 and switched seamlessly into another language to deliver the message again. The shuttle jarred slightly as they docked and Ippa waited for her row to be given permission to unbuckle. A man above her was too eager in his departure and sailed right into Ippa.

He smiled at her. "My apologies."

"It's fine." It was fine. It wasn't the worst thing to happen to Ippa over the past two days.

It took time to load passengers in shifts into the transition hall. When it was Ippa's turn, she dutifully navigated the handrails that guided her to the surface that would become the floor. Gravity initiated and Ippa slumped to the ground. She took another deep breath and went to find her bag. She had a feeling there were many deep breaths in her future.

Most of the other travelers got on a connecting flight headed to a much bigger port. One young man with a pencil-thin mustache immediately laid on the floor, made his bag a pillow, and was asleep within minutes. Ippa walked slowly around the outpost, her feet nearly dragging. At a secondhand shop that smelled of stale clothes, Ippa neatly and slowly refolded her Shou garments and traded them in. They fetched a good price (only fair because a good price was what she paid for them), and received in exchange three pairs of pants, four tunics, and a thick jacket. She still had her underwear, socks, and boots from home.

Ippa rolled up the last tunic, stowed it in her bag, and there it was: the end of her plan. She stood in front of the shop, wondering where to go next. For all the time she spent on the subject, she knew only two things: she was not welcome at The Shou, and she was not going home. She had some, but not much yurr. Most of her money was tied up in nonrefundable university fees, and she had no future prospects. Ippa wondered abruptly if the university would alert her parents that she had been expelled. Maybe she should send them a message. Or tell them she was out on assignment.

A blur of iridescent blue shot straight into Ippa's soft canvas bag and went tumbling over. Ippa stood, alarmed at the sudden disruption and peered down at a large amount of wriggling. Pencil-Mustache snorted loudly once, then rolled over, asleep.

At Ippa's feet, the blue ball unrolled itself into a furry body and four legs. The creature had a bandit stripe across its eyes and a thin, fur-covered tail. It was clearly a minkin. Ippa remembered studying the species's hair samples under a microscope at The Shou, but of course she had never had opportunity to meet one of the animoid species.

"Oh, I'm so sorry," Ippa said.

"You shouldn't stand in the walkway," the minkin blurted. She paced nervously around Ippa's bag as she sniffed it.

"Oh, of course."

"Anyone could trip." She ran her nose along the handle of the bag with such sincerity, Ippa wondered if she was about to chew on it.

"Oh, well yes, you're right." Ippa wished the minkin would move on. She didn't seem quite as upset as her words tried to make Ippa believe.

The minkin cocked her head to the side, to better see Ippa.

"Oh," the minkin said. "And oh. And oh again." She chuckled.

"Yes, well, excuse me." Ippa picked up her bag and turned left. Then right. She was suddenly paralyzed with fear. She spent her entire life working her way into the university, and now she didn't have enough of a life plan to tell her which way to turn.

"Are you a runaway?" the minkin asked.

"No. Of course not," Ippa snapped. "Besides, I am an adult. I could go anywhere I wanted and it wouldn't be running away."

"It looks like you're running away."

"Listen, I'm from the un—er, I'm going to rest here for a moment. I'm taking in the sights." Ippa wished the creature would move on so she could think clearly.

The minkin sat on her haunches next to Ippa and surveyed the outpost with her. Besides the secondhand shop, there was a food cart, a money exchange, several sleep capsules (clearly the second choice for Pencil-Mustache), and a few mundane supply stores. Her fur bristled, standing straight up. "You know, you should never lie to a minkin."

"What?" Ippa asked, panicked. She raced through her memory of the coursework they had done on Intelligent quadruped life, seeking some answer.

"It's true. If you lie to them, you have to give them your bag."

"What? Oh. Oh, get away, you nasty creature." Ippa jabbed at the minkin with her foot, not entirely sure if she was opposed to making contact. The minkin jumped out of the way.

"What do you have in there? Popcorn?"

"No, I don't have *popcorn* in my bag," she said. The Earth term tumbled uncomfortably from her mouth. "Why would I have *popcorn* in my bag?"

"Just a guess," the minkin replied and scuttled away.

Ippa knew of the volcano-dominated home planet of the minkins, but she knew nothing about their thought processes. The early years at the university focused on the physical, not the metaphysical. Ippa thought the minkin might stop to sniff the sleeping man's feet, but she scampered straight past and into an open vent.

Ippa's head shook of its own accord as she tried to understand what had happened. That some creatures were just rude beings was all Ippa could land on. She picked up her bag, went to the money exchange, and entered her account number. She was eager to be away from the minkin and anyone who had watched that little encounter. Checking her account was the only purposeful thing she could think of doing. She let the machine scan her retina. A small number appeared on screen, but it wasn't nothing. Ippa had worked as a coder between her acceptance and entry to The Shou.

The amount was nowhere near enough to take a grand traveling voyage and experience the many places she studied, something Shou students often did after graduation, but it could be enough to go somewhere. Some place in the galaxy.

A gut instinct hit Ippa so strong, she knew it was the only way. Ippa did not stop to perform a Sizco Benefit Analysis or write out a timeline of the plan.

She priced out a ticket, last stop, the Sol System.

Ippa was the closest thing to an expert on Earth besides her professors and Earthlings themselves. No one spent major funding or time on studying the plain little planet. Ippa knew books' worth of facts on other subjects easily as well, but working within any discipline more mainstream would be tricky. An expulsion from The Shou blacklisted her from every professional route she dreamed of. If she tried to get a placement on a reputable planet, they would contact the university for a reference. Earth was so remote, their systems so defunct...it could work.

Ippa's mind raced through the fledgling plan. She could visit and do some true research. Just because she wasn't at the university didn't mean she had to stop her studies. She would see the land and culture firsthand and do some original research. Then, she would go back to The Shou and donate samples and artifacts. Ippa paused and smiled for the first time in days. Maybe she would sell the samples to the university. There was a strong case for their addition to the biblioplaza. She could prove to Jinu and everyone else that a matter of paperwork wouldn't stop her from living and learning.

A small ray of hope shone for the first time since Ippa left Professor Jinu's office. She could do this. Had to. It was the only way to redeem herself.

She hit the accept button and purchased a one-way ticket to the Jupiter Station with the bulk of her personal funds. The transaction finished, Ippa expected she would feel relieved. Instead, a sick feeling welled up deep in her chest.

A short time ago, she was a student at the preeminent university in the galaxy with a bright future ahead of her as a scientist. Today, she was traveling to Earth.

# Chapter 11

D-68
Animoid Detention Center, Earth

Buzz and motion have become a way of life for Prisoner D-68. His nasal pads burn uncomfortably from long exposure to large amounts of metals and occasional wafts of chemicals he cannot identify. He has all but forgotten pain is not his snout's default state.

He lays in his iron cell. The humans bring him wilted leaves and half-molded roots but at least they smell edible compared to the human foods they eat down the hall. His nails grow thick and horny. It is vulgar and crude, but there is no help for it; he has nothing to cut them with. He lumbers back and forth in his cell to work his leg. He no longer greatly misses the platelet. Though he could tell one of his own kind it was taken by his captors, in his heart, it is as if he was born with it missing. Like his burning snout, his wounded leg is simply an everlasting part of him. He has been betrayed by his own body.

He hears their words and remembers: *leg, water, D-68*. But, unlike the learning of his own kind, these human things do not seep into the essence of him. They sit uncomfortably on the surface. There is no set place in his mind for the human words and actions to live in as the culture and ways of his own people do. Though he learns, he understands he has not always known.

There is a day when the vessel stops moving. It is a welcome relief.

He has been planning during the long journey.

As soon as he can, he will escape the creatures and run and hide. No more rest. He will get used to climbing and moving, and then he will travel in the wind direction. It will take a long time. D-68 knows that he has been traveling very fast, but he thinks that if he can get his strength back, he could run back in twice the time. It will be a long journey, but then, he will be home. The kits will be there. He can't believe anything else except that the kits will be there.

There is great commotion throughout the craft. Unsettling fresh air wafts its way through an open door, all the way back to D-68's cell. They whoop and cry out. He does not understand what this means, but he is on guard. The human voices leave.

All is quiet.

He waits for a long time. Humans he has never seen before come in. He can tell them apart if he gives careful attention to the limp, long bristles on their heads and the shapes of their noses. They put him through the old routine of restraint and slowly guide him out.

At the opening of the vehicle, he wishes to pause and assess what is ahead, but these creatures have no patience for him. The sky is a brilliant blue and the temperature is terribly cold and the air thin. He feels held down to the ground in a strange way. D-68 shakes in fear and one of the animals makes the honking noise they do when they find amusement.

It is a place where nothing looks like anything. White flecks fall out of the sky and D-68 shies away from them until there are too many. It is bitterly, impossibly cold.

Out of the metal craft, the burn in his nasal cavity lessens until they bring him to another metal vehicle, small but robust. Always at his back, his side, powering through his restraints, is the threat of a zap.

He feels chilled and weak but understands they are driving across the ground, not through the skies. D-68 does not wonder where they're going. He expects the rest of his life to be an eternity of driving in one vessel to another. Get out and be herded to the next craft, then drive again.

Instead, they stop at an enormous structure. The building is the size of the main cliff in his hamlet. It is not made with the red rock of his home but of seamless gray. It stands stark against the terrifying blue sky. His mind reels at the amount of time and skilled laborers it would take to build something of that size. He grows warier of his captives every day.

He is bodily restrained and someone removes the dressing from his wound. Dr. Jo is not there. It is a new human. His leg is finished bleeding and leaking, but it still aches without the supportive platelet. Two guards stand at attention while three humans work on him. He hears their words and remembers: *amputated, thigh, detention block.* He takes these words in and keeps them for himself. Not to be more like them, but to help him remember the time when he knew only one way of life. It is hard work, remembering, but more natural than letting this way of existing soak into who he is.

Afterward, he is led through a hall with many, many cells. A creature with a black-and-white striped body sits up when it sees D-68. It lets out a bellow and jumps to the bars with amazing speed. Short stubby digits grasp the iron bars with force and a wrinkled sack under the creature's neck inflates as it bellows again. Other creatures appear at their openings, hooting at him, laughing at him. One has big rheumy eyes set on the sides of its narrow head and a tongue that flickers. Another is thin but tall with a mess of hooked claws on the end of its arms. Some are small like humans or even smaller. None so big as him. They all call out to D-68. Though he can't understand all they say, they mock him.

D-68 is led to a quiet room and chained down. Electricity buzzes nearby. Not for the first time does he see the chain locks and think of his status as a toolmaker. However, he does not consider how a fellow craftsman might make these strange contraptions. He is only embarrassed that he used to take pride in his simple stone creations. The humans have taken everything from him. His home, his partner and kits, his own leg platelets. They are even shaping the very insides of him.

A massive creature enters. His attention sharpens. This is not a frail human, nor like those uncontrolled beasts in the cells. The creature is nearly as large as he is with thick matted hair that makes D-68's bristly knees look like smooth stone. D-68 tenses as he assesses who would win in a fight, sick as he is.

The other sits down. "I'm Jeb," the beast says. "I'm here to prep you for your trial. That's not what I do regularly, but they noticed, heh, that I'm an alien and you're an alien…and thought we'd get along."

The beast smiles like the humans. It sits comfortably like the humans. But it is its own thing. D-68 does not say anything. He wonders what else this ally of the humans could do to tear apart his life.

Jeb runs a large unkempt paw over his rounded face. "I've been following Linkos in the news since I arrived on Earth. They're so proud of their small-time mining operation. And the attacks…I think the Earthlings were sold a bad permit, but they can't see it and will never give up their right to occupy. I don't know what to tell you. You are in a lot of trouble. You killed a team member. Bad news anytime, but even worse right now because of the political tension. They're going to have a trial.

"A lot of people—Earthlings—want you dead outright. Exterminated. Humanoid aliens are more than enough for them. You and me? They call us animoids."

The hairy creature Jeb assesses D-68, then leans forward. "You don't understand a word of this, do you?"

Jeb growls, suddenly fierce, and D-68 sees how it would go down in a fight between them, him with his wounded leg.

"They were supposed to be teaching you the language on the spacecraft," Jeb says in frustration.

"Jeb," D-68 says.

Jeb nods in response. "My advice to you is learn to talk like them. These humans, they like to use a lot of words. I've even developed the habit while living here. They don't have a real translator on-planet for your language. Moreover, Linkos, what they call your language isn't in any of the translator devices we have. It's not even written down yet." There's a pause. "Is any of this getting through to you?"

Someone knocks on the door and Jeb turns.

D-68 sees Jeb is going to leave. "Help," he says in the strange language.

Jeb looks at him straight in the eye, and D-68 bristles instinctively as if a threat was made, as Jeb leaves the room.

Many sleep cycles later, D-68 is brought outside his cell.

He has been practicing words with one of the orderlies, a stern woman with gray hair. Early on he learned *food tray*, *off duty*, and then *shit*. The woman tried to take the last word away but D-68 kept it.

D-68's limbs are tethered and muzzled. There are several guards and D-68 is tired of these small creatures and their oversized power.

The group arrives at an outdoor area. D-68 shakes with chill. He sees new chains in the ground. Standing nearby is a long thin tube. D-68's sensitive pads tingle. They are going to wash him, chained to the dirt. In this terrible cold, every moment will be agony. It is an uncalled-for harassment.

He assesses the upturned soil and rock.

"Why are we bathing him now, the day before the trial? It's not going to cover up the smell. Or is that you, Freddy?" a woman with short red hair says.

The other guard responds. "Piss off. That hairy monster came yesterday with a bunch of Joint Council paperwork. 'Full washing while imprisoned is a guaranteed right for animoids.'"

The guards wrap him in the new chains and release the old.

He could almost smile like these little animals do. It is easy to feel that the chains do not go nearly deep enough to hold him there. The concrete they are imbedded in is frail, like them. But they are confident and once they have him chained and begin prepping, for once there is no electricity nearby. D-68 knows this is his moment, his only moment to get away. If he does not escape now, he will be taken back into the building with the electricity and the metal rooms.

D-68 wrenches his arms and legs and someone cries out. The chains on his arms break free of the ground. His ruined leg is too weak so he uses arm strength to break those chains too. The creatures turn their guns on him and yell—if only D-68 had known how they worked when the soldiers came to the hamlet. D-68 rolls sideways into the nearest small beast, the female, as someone fires. He snatches her gun. There is power in it, but D-68 cannot access it. He points it at the humans and that gives them pause.

D-68 backs to the wall, immense to the humans, but a plaything to him. He throws the gun at someone and they crumple to the ground.

He runs in the old way, on his arms over and up the side of the rocky wall. Guns blast behind him and D-68 jumps down. A terrible ringing sounds and D-68 runs. The creatures chase him. He cannot move quickly across this flat ground, bogged with wooden plants and brush. He shakes, breathless from the exertion after being shackled so long.

D-68 sniffs and senses what he needs. Rock. Underground air. They are almost on him. A shot grazes D-68, but he hardly feels it in his adrenaline. He pulls and scrapes at the rock and it crumbles under his hands. The stone gives a wail of death and reveals an opening into the ground. D-68 takes to it like a fish to water and digs and pulls himself forward. He leaves a good-sized hole behind him, but the humans do not come in. A bullet flies but hits rock. He warms as he accesses a chain of tunnels and digs and turns, hardly thinking about where he is going or if he will ever see the surface of the Earthlings' planet again.

# Chapter 12
## Hloban
### New Washington, WI, Earth

"Daddy," Obani said as he spun in the chair on his knees to look his father in the eye. "I *want* you to turn it *on*."

Hloban chuckled and looked up from the storage locker. "I don't think so."

The *Caneille*'s console was currently dark. Waquas had set the preliminary navigation course the night before and Hloban didn't want Obani messing anything up in the hours before departure. The pilot's seat dwarfed Obani's small frame, but he was used to coming whenever he needed to connect his son with something other than Earth-life. Obani was always either there or bouncing on the hideous Earth couch Hloban had bolted to the floor some years ago. There wasn't much to do on the ship—it had traveled far less than he imagined it would when he first bought it—but it was an escape for at least a little while. The *Caneille ES12* wasn't an A1 class craft by any means, but it was a place to think on the past and what could have been.

Which was why it felt wrong that strangers would arrive and

board in a matter of minutes. He had taken a call last night from a woman named Eeriva, her Australian accent taking him by surprise.

"Hello, Mr. Milson, I'll be the executive officer on this mission."

"Hloban's fine." Going by Loera's surname still felt weird. "If Secretary-General Cortez is still insisting on sending someone along, I guess there's not much I can do about it—"

"Not if you want space clearance."

"—but I hope you know what you're in for."

"Rest assured, I do."

It was a regular phone call so he couldn't see her expression, but Hloban could tell from Eeriva's voice and insistence she was used to being in charge.

"Patrick Wire will be captain on the journey and—"

"I'm the captain."

There was no hesitation. "Not according to this brief, you're not. Cortez's office was clear on the order of things."

As Eeriva went on about supplies, he fumed at the ever-increasing loss of control he was having over this mission.

Through the open air lock doors came the reedy buzz of an electric cart humming closer. Hloban descended the back ramp in time to see a staff member driving Adam, Keyad, and Amanda out in an open-air golf cart. Hloban would have been freezing on that ride, but Adam sat sprawled across the back seat, sunglasses on, curly black hair rippling softly in the wind like he thought he was a fucking rockstar. When Hloban was Adam's age, his planet had just blown up, and he was living in basically a closet in Joint Council housing as he scrambled to get the paperwork together to prove he was an endangered race and deserved a place on a planet.

The cart slowed and Adam hopped out before it stopped completely. He shot Hloban a toothy grin, then reached for a small hard-covered case and a soft backpack.

"Hloban! Great day for a trip!" Adam called.

Amanda raced up the ramp with Adam. Keyad was much more subdued and collected his own things.

"Clearance came through okay?" Keyad asked.

"Actually, Loera's there now making sure everything's moving along. I'm hoping we'll get to leave a few hours early." Rarely traveling for work herself, Loera was used to shepherding things along on her team's behalf. And, as an Earthling married to an actual alien, there was a sort of reverence thrust upon her by those who worked in off-planet facing sectors.

Keyad met Hloban's eyes. "I understand why you want to get moving, but a few hours aren't likely to change much."

Hloban shrugged more offhandedly than he felt. "Then again, it might."

They both turned at the quiet whiz of an electric truck. It pulled alongside the small cart and two people got out.

"Hullo the ship!" an older man called out.

A bolt of electricity ran up Hloban's back. Cortez's people. Was *that* the imposter captain? He was *ancient*. His face was lined, his hair was gray, and he looked so…so…spry.

With no qualms about his age, Patrick threw a heavy pack over his shoulder and vigorously shook Keyad's and Hloban's hands.

"Welcome aboard!" Patrick said.

Hloban bit his tongue at being welcomed into his own spacecraft when Eeriva appeared at Patrick's side. Stocky and sturdy all around, she had hair the color of an emerald. Hloban definitely hadn't pictured that over their voice call.

"I'm glad we can talk in person," Hloban started. "I understand the brief had a few discrepancies."

Patrick and Eeriva looked at each other before Patrick threw a heavy hand on Hloban's shoulder. "My boy, we've got winds to catch. Get the supplies loaded. We can talk everything through when we're on our way." He shouldered past and left Hloban behind in disbelief. Patrick spotted Obani at the top of the ramp and yelled, "My, my, my, look at the little space cadet."

"He's a good captain," Eeriva said with no-nonsense emphasis. She turned to unload supplies before Hloban could respond.

Just as he was about to head inside and straighten things out, Waquas appeared on foot.

"Good day to launch, you think?"

Hloban understood it wasn't a question. They couldn't get much better conditions. It was a clear blue winter day. Thank the gods there was no lake hurricane brewing over Lake Michigan. The last time that happened, Winslow was grounded for two days.

"Here, catch," Eeriva called.

Hloban stopped a metal barrel inches from his shins. He carefully maneuvered it up onto the ramp. Eeriva hustled past Hloban with two heavy sacks and unloaded them on the floor of the craft with a squat so deep it made Hloban's thigh muscles groan. Eeriva's gaze went to the loud floral pattern of the couch.

Patrick sat with Obani at the controls, earnestly discussing buttons with the preschooler.

Hloban stood the barrel upright and took a moment to really look at his son. Leaving Obani behind and leaving Loera with all the parenting duties for potentially months was a weight. It didn't matter that she had her parents or that they had a very well-funded preschool. She'd be the one to wake in the middle of the night to get Obani a cup of water just an hour before her own alarm rang for a virtual, multi-time-zone meeting.

As rushed as Hloban was over the past thirty-six hours, he took time to add new photos of the two of them to the digital frame in Obani's room. He also scheduled the delivery of a train conductor's hat to arrive in a week, right when Obani would realize Hloban was actually gone, not merely out at meetings. And the threat of never returning to his son…that was a wound in his mind he dared not touch.

There was commotion in the craft as everyone fought to get settled. Not only was the craft at capacity already with the passengers, but Amanda's and Obani's presence—and his loud narration of a space battle—made the space more cramped than it should be. Eeriva was loudly telling Waquas that the storage space was too small for all the canisters. Hloban sighed inwardly. Leave it to an Earthling to bring huge metal jugs on a J9-sized spacecraft. Hloban could only hope they had everything they needed. No way were they going to delay for Eeriva to go find a third spare fuse for the oxygenator or something. At least all the bodies were making the space warm.

Hloban spent a few minutes calming Amanda (Yes, there were only two bunks. No, her son wouldn't be sleeping on the floor for three months. Yes, they would all be on sleep rotations.) before going back outside, hoping for a glimpse of Loera.

He was rewarded with the sight of her in the distance, walking along the administration building toward a passenger crossing. There was no mistaking her confident walk. Though his heart was heavy at the thought of leaving her, Hloban smiled as he set out at a good clip to meet her. In the distance, an engine sputtered to life and another one rumbled above in the sky.

It was nearly five minutes before he met Loera. When she saw him, she slowed and pulled her scarf down from her nose and mouth. He tried to match her stride and gave her a bright smile.

"Hey, all good?"

"Sure, if using your company's reputation to strong-arm your way into advanced clearance for your husband's private vacation/rescue is fun."

"It's not a vacation/rescue. It's just a rescue." Hloban frowned that she would make light of Yaniqui being stuck in a human trafficking ring.

"No," Loera clarified in a tight voice, "'Vacation/rescue' is the official designation on your paperwork."

"It is?" Hloban asked, nonplussed. "Why would that combination possibly be an option on the paperwork?"

"Cortez's office sent over paperwork for expedited clearance on the grounds of it being a rescue, but the office of Immigration Services didn't want to give Adam clearance to leave, probably due to the very immigration language Cortez has been advocating for. Immigration Services insisted the trip be defined as a vacation to put a set time limit on when Adam has to return to Earth. They can't do that to the rest of you as noncitizens, but they can for Adam. Thus, the vacation/rescue."

Hloban pushed further, but it was clear Loera didn't want to talk about the fascinating ins and outs of space immigration paperwork. They walked in silence for a step.

"I know nearly everything's set up, but Hoban, I can't help but think all of this is too rash."

Hloban took a steady breath. "Eeriva and Patrick arrived with the supplies. You have to see this woman. I don't think she'd let us go if we were twelve grains of rice short of our last meal. Everything will go fine."

"It's not about all of that. What about when you get there? It's dangerous, and I can't for the life of me think why you'd risk your life—everything we have—to rescue this kid. Not even rescue, for a one-in-a-million shot at rescuing her."

A woman in a tight-fitting jumpsuit and thick pink coat ran past Loera and Hloban. Hloban waited until she was out of earshot before responding. He'd been having conversations with Loera in his head all morning, so the words came easily to him.

"There are things that I don't understand about life on Earth. And you ask me to trust you. Well, this is a Wea Saavian thing. I couldn't live with myself if I didn't go."

Loera rounded on him, stopping them both in their tracks. "When I say that, it's about wearing special pants to go skiing or—or not calling people in the middle of the night. Not putting your life at risk for a stranger."

"But that's the thing, Yaniqui is my family. If my planet was still habitable, I'd be living there with her. I thought she was dead—"

"So, that's what this is about? You think you've got a shot at your old life?" Loera was used to dealing deadly blows to the competition and her assistants alike—but always with a perky or at least neutral voice lest someone accuse her of being hysterical in the workplace. She nailed the very idea of an undercurrent and did so then.

"No. No, absolutely not." He took her arm in one hand and looked intently at her face. "Maybe we haven't talked enough about this, or rather I haven't shared enough with you." They were nearly at the *Caneille*, so Hloban pulled her toward a sunny spot on the spaceport apron.

"You know Wea Saavians have arranged marriages. When I was born, there was no one compatible. I'm older than Yaniqui so it wasn't until she was born that the arrangement was made."

Loera knew this indeed and had been lying in wait. "Yes, according to the placement of the *stars*! That's so nutso, Hoban."

He allowed a small smile. "If I try to see it from an outsider's perspective, I know it's strange. Just as strange as it is to me that everyone on Earth basically chooses someone at random to marry. The divorce rate is extremely high here and, from my perspective, if people stay married but aren't happy, what's the point?" Loera looked like she was about to protest his assessment, but he pushed on. "All I'm saying is while growing up, the arrangements seemed as natural as breathing air. It was the way things were done."

Loera scratched her eyebrow softly and dipped her eyes in the other direction. "So, you feel you still have a responsibility to this person."

"Yes," Hloban emphasized. "And not just because we were matched. She's the only other Wea Saavian we know of. Keyad is coming. Adam is probably not coming to help her, but he's still coming. Loera"—he took her hand in both of his—"I don't want Yaniqui to suffer at the hands of Akar and I don't want my entire race to die out."

Tears came.

"But *you* could die."

To both.

Hloban crushed Loera against his chest.

"Who would I be, if I didn't try?"

The entire venture was daunting. Dealing with Eeriva in close quarters. Spending months away from his son. Having Cortez breathing down his neck. Then actually rescuing Yaniqui from a gigantic, above-the-board, Joint Council-protected human trafficking operation. And then dealing with whatever came after that.

It wasn't that Hloban was unfamiliar with uncertainty or hard things. That'd been his entire existence between the time his planet had died and crash-landing on Loera's couch after a New Washington dinner-party-turned-bender.

When he woke the morning after the party, cans and stray plates still littered the coffee table and the room was thick with the scent of too many perfumes. Hloban woke with a smile. Family legend had it that that was just when Loera entered her living room to see if that weird alien guy was still there. She was touched he'd smiled so brilliantly upon seeing her in her satin-lined bonnet, mascara smeared under one eye.

What Hloban never brought up during those storytellings was that he woke up smiling from the most amazing dream. He had dreamed of Yaniqui. He could barely remember what happened, but he was more content than he'd ever experienced. Then, when he woke, there, looking down at him warily, was the most kick-ass woman he'd ever met.

One was there. One wasn't.

He never had to choose between them.

# Chapter 13

Lozen (*Lo-zen*)
The Catchment, WI, Earth

Lozen stared at the razor that would change her life. She tentatively pulled the blade along the hairs of her upper calf to see how it felt. It pricked and left behind a raw, I'm-that-much-more-naked feel. With lake water from her bucket, she tried again. A little smoother.

Lozen untied her black braid and combed through her hair with her fingers. Left to hang, it reached past her hips. She wet her fingers and worked them along the backside of her scalp, starting behind one ear and crossing the circumference of her head to the other side.

She picked up the razor and scraped sideways along her scalp. It didn't do anything. Lozen turned the blade around in her hand, placed it at the roots, and pushed softly up. Something loosened. She did it again, firmer.

Dark tangles fell to the ground, writhing masses cast off.

Lozen went over the wide stripe once with the blade, then touched it with her fingertips, one hand still holding the top half of her hair up. The shaved line felt matted, not clean-cut and bristly like Monte's.

Again and again she dragged the razor across her head, wetting her scalp in between strokes. Water trickled unpleasantly down her neck and back. Stray hairs fell into Lozen's collar and scratched her neck. It was hard looking at her hair on the floor. Her beautiful hair, part of her own body. It was a bigger deal for her than for Monte, whose hair ended at her chin. She exhaled through her nose and tried to feel detached from the lost pieces of herself.

A pinch stung Lozen and hot liquid pooled at her fingers. She squealed and threw the razor down on the swatch of fabric that covered half her dirt floor. She held her hands tightly over the cut and cursed.

When she brought them away, blood covered one hand, but the run of heat had slowed. Lozen scooped some of her bucket water into a dish and washed her hands in it. She would dump it outside later, after dark.

She decided she was done with the shave, hoped it was enough, and took two scraps of thin cardboard to sweep the pile of black hair together.

Lozen did not want to toss it outside as she did with her other scraps. First and foremost, Lozen did not want anyone to know she'd cut her hair. It was a complete secret. That was why she cut only a little bit in the first place. The other layers of her hair would cover it. Second—and this was something she pretended not to admit to herself—she once heard a story of magic performed on a man and the key ingredient of the curse was his own hair. Like all stories of curses, the man went mad, ate an entire paperback book, and died when his stomach clogged and burst.

It was ridiculous, but all the same, she placed the handful of hair under the corner of her sleeping mat. She would burn it later.

Lozen stretched her arms above her head, interlocking her fingers together when they met. She had finished her only task for the day.

She put on another pair of socks and grabbed her sandals from next to her pallet. They were the gray handout kind from some U.N. agency, much to the United States's chagrin. They were separating at the edges. Soon they'd flap when she walked so Lozen was already on the lookout for a different pair.

Lozen left her wash bucket—she would fill it with lake water when she dumped the now rust-tinged water—but picked up her drinking water bag, which was mostly empty. She pushed a hanging blanket out of the doorway and shoved a sheath of tin to the side and replaced it behind her.

Yesterday, the air was cold and full of large flakes of snow, but today it was bright with only a threat of true winter chill. Her aunt's stories told of winters piled high with snow and winds that blew like jagged flint, but Lozen was used to drastic changes in temperature during the winters. Snow came and went like a wolf searching for game.

A plastic bag full of plastic bags rolled by. Lozen punted her foot forward, but Uzzie was there first. He let out a rough yelp and kicked it back to his older brother, Jerramy, who kicked at it automatically.

"Hey, Lozen." Uzzie kicked the ball her way. Like any seven-year-old, he would share, but preferred to gift so his friends remembered who had spent an entire day collecting and rolling plastic bags into a ball.

Lozen caught it with her foot and punted it to Jerramy. "How's it, Jerramy?"

Jerramy and Lozen kicked the ball quickly back and forth and Uzzie charged between.

Uzzie laughed. "That's great, guys," Uzzie said. "You're a real team. Okay, my turn now."

"I haven't seen your friend Monte for a while," Jerramy said, kicking the ball past Uzzie again. He smiled and a dimple appeared.

Lozen wished for one of those. She covered the smile she couldn't help give back.

"That can't be true," Lozen said. "She's here all the time. You're just never here." Lozen could already visualize the expression Monte would have when Lozen reported back that Jerramy asked about her.

Mama Teresa came around the corner.

Lozen wanted to continue the conversation for Monte's sake, but Jerramy and Uzzie were already disappearing.

Mama Teresa used to be just plain Teresa. At least, when anyone risked addressing her.

Then, one day, a hang-about named Tomi kicked the tin wall of her house. The wall fell and upended a bucket of hootch that spilled across her dirt floor, no longer drinkable. Teresa rushed out and attacked Tomi in retribution.

Lozen was napping that day when she heard Tomi's yowls. She came in time see Teresa whack Tomi's face with a broken brick.

That was harsh, even for Teresa.

Tomi crouched on the ground, crying, holding her nose, and shielding herself from Teresa's kicks. There was no way Lozen was going to jump in. Teresa had fifty pounds on her.

A tall man named Gerald came running down the path and pulled Teresa off Tomi. The brick fell to the littered ground and Teresa turned to bite Gerald.

Gerald held her back easily with his long arms and said, "Hey, Mama Teresa, it was time to turn over a new leaf anyway." Mama Teresa picked up the brick and swiped at Gerald, to show what she thought of that idea, but he plucked it out of her withered hands.

Mama Teresa advancing, Uzzie went into his large family's shack and Jerramy smiled at Lozen and set off on his own. Lozen avoided making eye contact with her aged neighbor and walked in the other direction. She wrapped the cord on her water bag around her wrist.

Every few steps lay a new shack made of tin or plywood, with items and bundled children with running noses spilling out into the worn pathway. She took a left turn, stepped over a rubbish heap that appeared yesterday, and followed the meandering path forward. One of the good things about the winter cold was it kept the smells down, even on mild days.

Those that lived directly around Lozen were displaced Earthlings, like herself, but about half the Catchment was made up of bona fide aliens, straight from outer space. Some looked like biological Earthlings. Others passed for Earthlings, but you felt a little uneasy looking them in the face. There was something different about them: facial features a smidge too far apart, or you suspected they had extra teeth. But they were still humanoids.

There on the path was a little four-footed animoid. It ran about the humanoid side of the Catchment, tolerated because it reminded everyone of a cat. Lozen liked to chat with him every once in a while.

"Hi, Lozen," he said, pausing to sniff the air. "It's going to snow tonight," he called over his shoulder.

He had shiny blue fur that was unheard of on Earthling animals. Lozen knew of more than one plot to capture and skin the animal, but none of the plans were ever pulled off successfully. The animal was a trickster, like Coyote.

The real animoid aliens were on the north side, farthest away from the lake. And stranger than extra teeth or a talking fur ball.

Scrupulously, Lozen tucked a finger under her hairline and ran it along the stripe, feeling for the raw nick and enjoying the smooth feel of her own scalp. Her long top layers of hair completely covered the shaved patch, but still, she felt like everyone knew it was there.

Lozen approached the busy water pump and got in line. The water was purely for drinking and you could fill your government-issued water bag only once a day. Around Lozen, those that finished collecting water gossiped and traded small items.

Since she was fourteen years old, Lozen had lived alone, so she had been collecting her own water every day, save during the long drought. Before that, her aunt had instilled the habit in her of collecting water first thing in the morning.

Just before her turn, Lozen lifted her bag up to her lips. She did not like to finish her water bag until she was sure she would have more clean water in hand, something else her aunt had taught her. It was hard for Lozen to drain the last of the bag. She tipped it and took care to keep her lips tight, but water dribbled down her chin. Lozen wiped it with her sleeve.

She filled her bag at the pump and headed toward her next stop of the day, the handout station. They gave only enough food for a day and for that, Lozen had a pile of small plastic tokens to trade. She had wondered more than once why they didn't hand out larger quantities of loath, the ground meal wrapped in sealed plastic bags that wound up discarded everywhere.

The dirt road between the water pump and the handout station was one of the widest in the Catchment, but busy and still lined by homes. An argument broke out from one shelter that was part tent. A baby wailed and stopped when someone cooed to it. Kids darted in and out, mixed races and species playing with each other. It always seemed easier for them.

Someone brushed up against her.

"Lozen."

She turned, already recognizing Monte's voice.

"Did you do it?"

Lozen shook her hair out slightly and covered part of her mouth with her hand when she smiled. She covertly removed the blade from the band of her pants and hid it from view while she gave it back to Monte.

"The station's not open, if that's where you're headed," Monte said.

"That's the second time this week."

"I have something for you though, from Charla. She gave everyone in the…" Monte paused, searching for the right word, "group one of these." Monte leaned close into Lozen, just two girls chatting on the street. Lozen was fit, but Monte was truly slender, something Lozen was acutely aware of when they were physically close. Monte slid a heavy object into Lozen's pants pocket, the weight settling against her leg. "Don't take it out here."

Monte linked arms with Lozen and the girls wandered more slowly to the handout station to see what was going on. It was a good place to people watch.

"Did you meet up with Dan last night?" Monte asked while they walked.

"It was terrible," Lozen said. "I called him Dan-the-Man."

Monte laughed, made eye contact with Lozen, and laughed harder. She tucked her short hair back, still wheezing.

Weeks ago, Lozen and Dan drunkenly fooled around by the shore one night. It was fun, but the repeat had not gone well.

"I don't think I'm interested," Lozen told Monte. It was partly true. Lozen wasn't interested in pursuing anything else, but not because Dan wasn't likable. She was the unlikable one. Sober, Dan could not seem to forget about her cleft lip. His eyes traveled to it repeatedly while they talked and he was reluctant to pick up where they had left off when Lozen leaned into him.

Lozen didn't pause to wonder if Monte guessed the truth. She moved the conversation forward before Monte could ask for details. "Jerramy, however, seems interested."

Monte's face froze.

"In you, silly," Lozen said. "He asked about you this morning." The idea of someone preferring her to Monte was laughable.

A thundering roar filled Lozen's ears and she staggered, dropping hard upon the ground. The earth shook. Her hands prickled with pain from the gravel ground. Lozen barely noticed. A wave of heat overtook her.

Lozen went dumb. Why was it suddenly so hot? Was it the weather? Was something big finally happening? Her pulse raced in the side of her throat. Images of radiation-burned skin ran through her head.

Lozen tried to right herself. Dust streaked one side of Monte's face.

There was a raging blaze where the handout station once stood.

Monte stood and gave Lozen a hand up.

They pushed their way through a gathering crowd of Catchment residents. Terrified kids cried and older ones pulled them away, back toward a safer place. Lozen saw a little boy with dusky blue skin lying on the ground. Blood seeped from his head.

"Oh my gods, I was here," Monte whispered. "Just before I saw you."

People gathered around the child, faint with life. Some of the crowd started pulling rubbish away from the growing circle of flames. One family tore at their makeshift siding, trying to disassemble their house before it caught fire. Lozen felt a mad urge to laugh as they crawled over their home like ants. A woman vigorously kicked dirt onto the smaller flames and others followed suit.

Monte jerked into action, grabbing Lozen's hand. They joined in kicking dirt. Open flames scorched Lozen's face, making her skin tight. She stepped back to pull off her outer sweatshirt and held it bunched loosely over her mouth and nose to protect from the ash and scorching air.

As much as they beat and kicked at the fire, the group could put out only the smallest flames on the outskirts. The structure itself blazed too hot and too high.

Monte pulled on Lozen's arm. "Let's get out of here. The regulators will be here soon."

An old man nodded. "They don't care about much, but this they'll want to see."

With the fire in the distance, they took short pulls from Lozen's fresh water bag. Monte shook out her short hair and wiped her neck and face with an ashy hand, smearing black and gray along her sweaty brow.

"I gotta go," Monte said. "Are you okay?" She said the last word as if it were cut in two, drawn out to the point of a nonsensical slur. She took a breath and calmed herself. "Are you okay?"

Lozen gave her friend a shaky hug. "You do what you have to. I'll be with you soon."

Monte reminded her of the night's meeting place and then headed south.

Alone, Lozen continued on her own to her house. She shifted aside the tin door and lifted the blanket. She made for her pallet, exhausted. When she hit the ground, she felt a hard shape in her pocket and remembered Monte placing something inside earlier. She pulled out the item—an apple, bruised on one side.

Lozen ate the apple, all but the stem, and lay back, exhausted. Her red, smoke-ridden eyes shut immediately.

A rat scratched near Lozen's head. She swatted the rodent away and it escaped through a hole at the bottom of a wall. Lozen had recently finished collecting enough nails to pull canvas over the hole, but now the material was chewed through.

Late afternoon sun spilled through cracks, casting a reddish glow about her. Lozen was groggy and surprised she slept so long. She took a careful drink of water. Already the night chill was coming on. She had to get going if she was going to make it in time. She grabbed her ugly purple coat from the rafters of her small house and tucked it under her arm. Outside, a trail of smoke lingered in the sky, thankfully thin. Lozen felt the retroactive pull of panic. She never should have fallen asleep after the blast. What if the fire had spread? Her pulse quickened at the thought and she had to reminded herself that it hadn't.

Lozen walked briskly along the narrow pathways in the direction of the Great Lake. When dirt turned into silt, she left her socks and sandals on the sand, rolled up her pants, and waded into the cold water. From the beach, she overheard a few small girls plotting to catch a seagull for dinner.

As huge as it was, the lake wasn't good for drinking anymore, but it was fine to wash in. Lozen scrubbed her face, feet, hands, and arms. Her skin shivered and chilled where she splashed brisk water on it. She wet her hands again and ran the water through her long black hair. The smoky smell of fire awoke, freshened by the water. Her hands came away dark and she repeated the process. Lozen shook everything thoroughly and squeezed out her hair, careful not to expose the small strip of new nakedness.

With the setting sun to her back, Lozen stood, stretching her arms and staring across the persistent waves. She thought far back to when the travelers came down from the sky to settle and grow and then even further back to the day the travelers came across the sea to build and take, and finally back to the time when the shoreline was healthy and her people lived on the land.

The land was now fully settled—ships flew overhead, the space elevator glinted in the far distance—but the lake was steadfast. It was broken, polluted beyond drinkability, but it had outlasted those who destroyed it. Lozen didn't have much to connect her to the traditions of her people, but she would always remember the stories her aunt told her about the small Nibinabe and the powerful Nambi-za that lived in the lake.

The sky was darkening and she had a long walk ahead of her. She pulled her thick jacket on and zipped it up, the zipper catching and requiring a short struggle.

She kept the sun to her right and slipped out of the loosely fenced Catchment, as instructed by Monte. The ground was hard dirt, picked clean and packed down by foragers, that gradually evolved to small brush, then trees.

Lozen scratched her shaved hairline, mindful of the tiny scab, and thought about the explosion as she walked. Flames and burning heat surrounded by thousands of people. That was one of the greatest fears within the Catchment: a fire, wind whipping it out of control until nothing was left, not even anyone to see it.

There had been much discussion about creating firebreaks, so that if one area went down, the others wouldn't be subjected to the same fate. Most liked it in theory but deciding where to put the gaps was near impossible. There was too much possession over certain areas. Everyone wanted to clear land in someone else's territory.

Lozen walked a long time, but she didn't tire. Everyone was used to walking in the Catchment.

The sun graciously lowered itself to make way for the moon. The air grew cold and brittle after such a warm day. The winter wind was back. It chilled her damp feet. A giant clump of snowflakes drifted past. Lozen looked up and was surprised to see the sky laden with them, though she shouldn't have been—the little fur ball told her they would come.

The cliff line was far from the crowded Catchment, but Lozen supposed there was no place for a secret among all those people. Once she hit the rocks, she turned right and followed along.

At last, she saw a tentative light come from a fissure in the cliff. The amber glow grew as she moved through the last of the forest trees. Though Lozen expected to find it there, miles away from the Catchment, fear crept over her. She didn't know what was going to happen inside the cave. Despite the cold air, her neck was slick with sweat.

The snow settled thickly under Lozen's plastic sandals. Inside, beyond numerous footprints and out of the bitter gusts, two women held torches in the stone recess. Lozen touched the uneven skin of her lip briefly before stepping into the fullness of their light. The stagnant cold of stone and abyss greeted her, but at least there was no harsh howl of wind.

Lozen took a string out of her pocket and tied up half her hair to show the stripe that matched her sisters-to-be. One tall woman nodded her forward and they walked into the dark cave, lit only by flame.

"I've never felt so cool in my life," Lozen said. She shrank back, certain she shouldn't have admitted that.

"Yeah, I'm cold too," one of the women said, missing Lozen's confession.

The women led Lozen deeper into the rock belly, twisting and turning through the pathways. More than once, her foot slipped. A *whoosh* of air passed over Lozen's head; a bat on its way to hunt. Lozen looked behind—nothing but dank black—and realized she might not be able to find the way out on her own.

A whisper of a voice brushed Lozen's ear, but neither of the women had spoken.

Moving past a twisted column of rock, they reached a large cavern. Darkness masked the edges, but in the center, a large group of women stood in a loose half circle. Lozen saw gray masses of supplies behind them but couldn't identify them in the dark. She wondered if any of the crates held weapons and felt suddenly too cold. Everyone turned to look at her, the sentinels standing on either side.

"You wish to be the Karma upon this world, Lozen?" a clear, high voice asked her.

Lozen turned toward the woman who spoke from the side of the grouping. *That must be Charla,* she thought, *the leader and sender of the apple.* She had long box braids, half piled on top of her head. If the woman turned, she guessed she would see a shaved arch on her skull. The darkness obscured much of her, but Lozen could see well enough to watch Charla assess her. She looked over Lozen's tired clothes and rested her eyes on the cleft lip.

Lozen fought the urge to cover the bottom part of her face and spoke as solidly as she could, "I am Karma." Over the past few days, she had rehearsed the simple words many times in her head, but didn't say it aloud in the Catchment for fear of being overheard. Surrounded by stone, with new words, Lozen didn't sound like herself.

"And will you keep our secrets, sister? For they are many."

"I will make the secrets my own and keep them until death."

None of the men in the Catchment knew about the Karmas. Lozen certainly didn't know until Monte confessed a few days ago that she had joined the most elite and secretive society within the Catchment. Lozen could not see her friend in the torch-lit cavern.

"Then prove what you are. We rectify wrongs in the Catchment.

The three bosses as they call themselves—Lin, Jimson, and Pellor—care more about money and personal vendettas than keeping families safe. No one will help us, so we will help ourselves.

"Your assignment is to find the fire culprit and bring him to justice. He tore food away from our families and killed two young ones and an old man."

Lozen's heart sank. She knew there would be a challenge, an initiation, to join the Karmas, something to prove she held the interests of the Catchment close. But this was so much more than she expected. Part of her had hoped the group was together just for jokes. A fun little club of women.

*No,* Lozen realized, *this was very real.*

"To succeed in your initiation, find him and give him justice," Charla said.

"Him?" Lozen asked.

The woman smiled, white teeth shining, her face almost gone in the dark of the cavern.

"It's always a him."

# Chapter 14

Adam
In Transit

A small transmitter beeped next to Adam's ear and he opened his eyes easily. He got so much sleep on the *Caneille* that he suspected he was awake in all but consciousness long before it was time to roll out of the bunk. Captain Patrick slept in the other bunk and was scheduled to for another four hours. Adam stepped down on quiet cat feet and stretched.

Adam didn't bother to change clothes. He patted down his black hair—it was two weeks past his usual haircut—and looked at the digital communications board. His personalized schedule said his half hour for breakfast would start in five minutes. After that, he was scheduled for a vague maintenance and cleaning session for four hours.

He'd be early for breakfast.

Adam shut the door softly behind him and went to the bolted-down table to eat his meal bar and water packet. He broke the seal on the airtight container of bars. In addition to a soft *woof,* he was greeted by a pungent, tangy smell. His dad was in charge of food preparation and added fish oil to most of the bars. Good for brain health, he always said. Adam chewed woefully.

Waquas was at the ship's controls, his green skin gone funny in the light of the console. Eeriva typed on her tablet. Aquaponics grew along one wall and the rest of the walls were made up of metal panels and secured cabinets, so Adam stared out the nearest porthole.

The ship—*spacecraft*, only Earthlings called them ships—was the one Hloban had originally flown to Earth. It had only five spaces: the mains that consisted of the cockpit and open living area, the dormitory, a broad hallway off the mains that led to the air lock doors and boasted a number of cabinets, a tiny exercise room, and an even tinier bathroom. It was one of the smallest models to have Lightspeed+ capacity. At the outskirts of the Sol System, the spaceship would alight within the travillion, the negative matter entry point, and antimatter fuel would boost them to Lightspeed+.

Patrick had utilized the ship's software to assign duties and schedules. He had put Adam in charge of maintenance and cleaning, but no one had time to train him on any equipment. He spent much of his time trying to clean the bathroom without water. Adam wasn't even allowed to change the filter on the oxygen machine. He argued changing the filter *was* cleaning, but his father pointed out that it was part of the most important piece of equipment on the ship. On the spacecraft.

A shriek came from the sleeping quarters.

*Finally.*

Adam threw the rest of the disgusting bar in his mouth and brushed his hands on his pants.

Once in the bunk quarters, Adam had trouble making sense of what he saw. Patrick wasn't facedown as he usually slept. Hloban had rolled him over. Patrick was stiff, blue in the face, and his skin was shiny.

"What's going on?" Waquas asked from the console. No one answered him.

"Oh no," Eeriva moaned, suddenly at Adam's side.

They all turned to look at her. After all, she and Patrick had arrived together, sent by Cortez's office. Adam couldn't imagine her bawling and writhing on the floor, but he prepared for it anyway.

"What are we going to do with him?"

"Eeriva! 'What are we going to do with him?' You can't say that over a dead body."

"Why not, Hloban? You just did."

"What—what killed him?" Adam stuttered. "I mean, he was fine." Adam blinked again in case he was misunderstanding things. His arms jittered.

Eeriva looked sideways at Adam, "He was eighty-two years old. What didn't kill him? They almost didn't let him go, you know."

"Who?" Adam asked.

"His kids. But Commander Vera insisted because of his experience and there was nothing his family could do about it."

"Shit, I didn't know he had kids." Adam pictured sweet little toddlers.

"Again, the man was eighty-two years old. I think they live in one of the tech cities in the plains." Eeriva stood silently for a minute. "All right, what are we going to do with him?"

"Eeriva," Hloban groaned.

"Listen, I'm not heartless and I care—cared—for him more than any of you." Eeriva dug her fingers into her hair and shook it out, definitively looking away from the body. "I was on Patrick's crew the first time I went up. He requested me specifically for this mission because he knows I know protocol and protocol says we can't keep him here. He's going to bloat and liquefy before we get to the girl."

That triggered Hloban to repeat his far oft-used line, "We're not stopping." He had been resolute on that point since they left Earth.

"So much for sentimentality, Hloban."

"We'll have to eject him with the waste," Adam spoke up. "We have to release before we boost anyway."

At last, Adam's dad said, "I guess it's better to do it while he's in the solar system, as close to home as possible. His family's not going to be happy with us though."

The others drifted back to their duties as Adam and Eeriva wrapped the body in a sheet of clear plastic. The body didn't smell, but Adam breathed through his mouth anyway. The limbs were heavy and flaccid as Adam moved them into place. Adam wondered if they should put Patrick's shoes on. Patrick's face loomed, distorted through the wrapper as they carried him to the mains. Eeriva moved as if she hauled dead bodies every other week. Adam was the one struggling with the man's weight and bulk.

While waiting for whatever was next, Adam washed his hands—a real washing with liquid soap and slightly more water than he should have used. He pictured himself dying of thirst in the middle of nothingness, but he couldn't stop washing where Patrick's wrapped head rolled against his forearm.

"Adam, put the food containers away," Eeriva barked. "What if we need the tabletop in an emergency?"

At first, due to Eeriva's accent, Adam had mistakenly treated her commands as less intense than her words implied. Australians sounded so casual and she was always saying things like "woop woop." Now he knew better. Adam dried his hands. "Eeriva, how many voyages have you been on?"

Eeriva stopped charging around the hold, doing whatever it was she did. As she paused, Adam saw a slice of musty blond at the roots of her teal hair.

"This is my thirteenth journey and will be my sixth boost."

She had seen more of the universe than 99 percent of Earth combined.

Adam cleared his throat. "I think I should do it. I should release Patrick into the great unknown."

Eeriva rolled her eyes. "You want me to teach you how to use the releaser."

"Yes, so I can help Patrick. I was there with him when it happened."

"Then maybe you should have stopped it."

"I was sleeping. You said he was going to die anyway!"

"Adam, I understand," Eeriva said and touched Adam on the shoulder, something Adam was certain came not from instinct but from a ship manual on calming crew members in times of crisis. "But we don't want to botch this. I knew him from before and I'm acting captain now. I should do it."

Adam hoped Hloban didn't overhear Eeriva refer to herself as captain, or at least that they could put off fighting until Adam got to use the releaser. He tried again, "I can't help if I don't know anything. What if something else happens? What if someone"—Adam didn't want to say *died*—"gets hurt and I can't even perform basic functions on the ship?"

Eeriva thought about that. Adam could see the idea taking hold. *Yes.*

"I'm not the one who told you that you could come, but okay. You can help."

Adam visualized the process. "Okay, so we just…we'll put his body in the waste area and remove the locks?"

"No. I'm not heartless; we'll do a service first."

Adam organized Patrick's things into a small bag for his kids—grown-up, probably advanced-in-age-themselves adult kids—to have when they got back to the ground, but in the meantime, he placed them at Patrick's feet.

"I sent a notice to Winslow," Eeriva said as everyone lined up in front of the body. "They'll contact his family." She turned to Adam. "I believe you were with Patrick when he died?"

"Uh, yeah, but we were both sleeping."

"And you're also going to be disposing of the body?"

Adam stayed silent. He knew where this was going.

"Ad-am, Ad-am," Waquas started.

Adam jerked, stung with outrage. "Oh my gods. I'll speak. Let's have some respect, people."

Adam turned to face the group. "It's too bad Patrick died because he was a hero. He said he'd help despite how difficult he knew the mission would be for him. His kids will miss him, but they didn't see him at his finest, traversing the solar system. Rest in peace, Patrick."

"Here, here," Eeriva said over the top of something illegible from Waquas.

Everyone went back to their duties. Adam marveled at how easy they were with Patrick's death. Perhaps on voyages someone is expected to die and Patrick wasn't a bad choice as far as things went.

Adam and Eeriva lifted Patrick once more. The thick plastic

sheeting crinkled and the slipping and sliding planted Patrick's head against Adam's chest. Together they waddled across the room, down the only hallway of the ship, and back to the storage areas by the air lock doors.

Eeriva lowered his feet into the receptacle. Adam grunted, holding on to the torso. He had pictured gently lowering the body in and reclining it to a dignified position, but he couldn't quite reach the bottom.

"Now what?" Adam asked.

"It's up to you, mate. You're the one in charge here."

His arms hurt. There was nothing left to do except to drop the body. It fell with a *whump* and a crackle of plastic. Adam bent over and saw Patrick's body lying across a pile of small compostable bags of human fecal matter, already stripped of their nutrients, ready to float in the vastness of space until they flung themselves into the sun or burned upon entry in an atmosphere.

Eeriva stood in front of the small control panel. "OK, now we enter the security code. I cannot stress enough that this is only for approved usage."

"I'm not going to go flush happy."

"No, you're not, because the code changes every twenty-four hours."

Adam struggled to find words. "So…you not only think that I'd abuse the power of the releaser, you think that I couldn't hold out for more than a day?"

"Every ship changes their code every twenty-four hours." She muttered, "How can you be out here and not know this?"

That last comment stung Adam. "What are you going to do? Memorize a new six-digit code every day?"

"Yes, of course, that's what I'm going to do. Because it's regulation. As in…rules." She took a breath. "Sometimes on long trips, people go a bit crazy. Well, really crazy. It's best if the essential details are split up among a few well-trusted people."

Adam sensed juicy details. "When you say crazy…?"

"I mean violent disagreements about rations and love triangles that end with murder-suicides."

As easy as pie, Eeriva shifted topics and gave Adam the directions, recited the precious six numbers, and told him to press the gray button. A soundless *whoosh* that rang within his bones shook the ship. *There goes Patrick,* Adam thought, and tried to reorientate his inner dialogue into something respectful that fit the occasion.

There was another shriek.

*What the hell? Were they not all adults here?*

"What did you do? What did you do that for?" Eeriva said.

Hloban and Keyad came running, one half-asleep and bleary-eyed and the other with sticky hands held in front of him.

"You stupid, stupid boy."

"What's going on back there?" Waquas shouted from the front. No one answered him.

"What the hell," Adam said. "*Stop* hitting me."

Eeriva was furious. She flared her nostrils and her eyebrows made a deep crease. The side of her neck throbbed. If it wasn't directed at Adam, it would have been funny.

"You pressed the wrong button."

Adam did an anxious double take at the control panel. *No, there was the gray button, right there.*

Eeriva gestured wordlessly to an identical round one on the opposite end.

Hloban groaned. "He flushed the wrong system. Is that what happened, Eeriva?"

"Yes. We were using one of the dispensers as a storage container for the food that didn't fit in the main cabinets."

Adam panicked. "What was food doing in there at all? And why *the fuck* wouldn't you have told me?"

Eeriva started arguing, "I told you which button to press, you weren't listening—"

"You said 'Push the gray button, Adam' and that's what I did." He threw his hands up in the air.

"No, I said the gray button on the left!"

"I can't believe you didn't tell me—"

"Adam, stop. We had to use the smaller dispenser because we brought so many supplies. This ship is designed for only six and we were planning on bringing a seventh person back with us," his dad said. He licked his lips. "We're going to have to stop for food and water."

Hloban spoke with icy conviction, "Absolutely not—we don't have time. Yaniqui doesn't have time."

Everyone moved away from the panel and Adam asked, "What about Patrick? He's still here, right?"

Eeriva aggressively walked up to the panel and did the complex button sequence in seconds. The green light blinked and she waved exaggeratedly toward the gray button on the left. Adam pushed it; they heard the soundless bone-chilling *whoosh* for the second time.

Adam felt like shit all the next day. He hadn't wanted to mess up Patrick's final moments with humanity. He hadn't wanted to flush out their food. And he definitely didn't want to be punished with hours of collecting dust particles and dead skin cells with a vacuum the size of his hand.

His dad and Eeriva were sleeping. Waquas was in the gym and Hloban was at the console, keeping an eye on the navigation set to autopilot. Up on one of the screens was an article.

Adam vacuumed the vent over and over again above Hloban's left shoulder as he read along with Hloban. Akar Enterprises was the business of an investor's dream. It made handful over handful of money acquiring and selling rare beings. Adam tried to imagine being pinned in a position like that—freedom gone, potential owners circling.

"Do you think she gave herself up to them?"

Hloban startled at the sound of Adam's voice. The hum of the tiny vacuum had lulled both of them. Adam clicked it off.

"I said, 'Do you think she sold herself to them?'"

"Yaniqui? No, never."

"She was pretty young when Wea Saa died though. Maybe she had no choice."

Hloban shook his head in irritation. "You don't understand."

Adam shrugged his shoulders in challenge.

Hloban took a breath and leaned back in his chair. "Wea Saa was an incredibly peaceful place, but everyone had a sense of looming threat regarding anything outside the planet. When you're somebody who has what others want, it's too easy to imagine the onslaught of desire and greed. It's drilled into Wea Saavian heads: be wary of others."

"My dad doesn't talk about it."

"You never think of it, Adam?"

"What?"

Hloban turned around more in his chair to watch Adam's expression. "You can heal only yourself, but has it ever occurred to you that you could be captured and forced to reproduce in hopes that your offspring would be a girl? Hell, with a bit of your sperm, a trafficking company like Akar could artificially grow hundreds of babies. They could ditch the males, or keep some as insurance, but sell the females as healers for basically however much money they wanted."

"Shit."

"Yeah, 'shit.' And that's just one scenario."

Adam didn't say his dad never broke it down for him like that. He didn't want Hloban to stop talking because he felt he had to protect Adam too.

"So, if it's really just you, me, my dad, Obani, and Yaniqui…"

"And Yaniqui's mom, Nica. They were off-planet at the time of the solar flare—it was one of the reasons why I continued looking for her, but I always assumed things went wrong for them way back then. I remember being terrified of Nica. She would have drilled this threat into Yaniqui and forbidden her from doing anything to give them away. So, no, I don't think she offered herself up to Akar."

"So, if Akar has Yaniqui, where's her mom?"

# Chapter 15

### Yaniqui
### In Transit

Yaniqui woke stretched across soft lavender sheets. She didn't remember a time when she woke without opening her eyes to the grumbling of her mother, a whining baby, or some immediate task that needed to be taken care of. For her entire adult life, her morning routine had been the same: wrap herself in the thick waist wrap regardless of the temperature, brush out and tie back her curls, splash water on her face from the communal bucket, eat a bland breakfast, and head to the fields. The only bits of excitement came when she and Sario ducked out of breakfast early to scheme. No. She wasn't ready to think of Sario yet.

    She opened her eyes and simply lay there. She had taken a chance and found a life of luxury. Eventually she stirred and sat up in the bed, the covers still pulled up to her camisole. The cooler air outside her nest brushed against her sleep-warmed skin. She considered what to do first. Eat? Bathe? Skip both and dress? She could do anything. Be anyone. It felt like freedom.

    Yaniqui went in the—what did they call it? The W.C.?—and

relieved herself. She gave a long look at the shower stall and reminded herself of what the attendant had said last night.

"You'll want to turn that on and get in immediately," the woman said, eyeing Yaniqui. "Put your clothes in the drop bin. Those ragged things are done. Your showering quota is eleven gallons every day. The lights will signal when you're almost out, so make sure you rinse in time." The steady woman had closed the shower door after demonstrating the knobs. It was clear she had orientated many people before Yaniqui.

Yaniqui was afraid of the officially dressed woman with cheeks as smooth and blemish-free as polished stone, but curiosity peppered her like a persistent mosquito. She blurted, "And I can shower every day?"

"Yes, ma'am," the servant replied, surprised, but polite. "Akar Enterprises wants to ensure your utmost comfort and well-being."

Well, if Akar cared that Yaniqui's hair was clean, it was the least she could do.

Once the woman was finished giving the tiny tour and had left, Yaniqui investigated more thoroughly. She had stripped her clothes and threw them away when she was sure there were fresh garments in the room. Like the woman suggested, Yaniqui got in the shower immediately, before she could soil any part of the stunning guest room.

Comfort overcame her quickly as steam seeped into her pores and she lathered a measure of soap on the top of her head. In minutes she was washed and stood under the pouring water until the lights glowed blue, gradually deepening in color until no more water came out.

Drying off, she caught her reflection in the mirror and examined her face, but it took a moment before she realized the full implications. There she was. She saw her body for the first time, as the women in the labor camp did. Curling black hair to her shoulders, more often a snarl than not, powerful upper arms from working in the fields, rounded breasts she held in the dark so often, and a thin waist above a mass of dark hair. Yaniqui turned around and waggled her buttocks in the mirror. A laugh broke out. It was with a measure of cautious optimism that she dressed in soft pajamas and fell asleep quickly.

On her first morning with Akar Enterprises, Yaniqui considered that she could shower again, even after having showered just the night before. No one was going to tell her not to. It was the luxury of fairy tales.

She spent some time in the bathroom rubbing polishes and tonics into her face and body until her skin glowed with good health. The soft olive tones radiated hydration and rest for the first time.

In the main room, Yaniqui dressed in a style of clothing she'd only seen in ads among news stories on Fra Yu's Loscroll. She pulled on dark wide-legged trousers made in a thick, almost scratchy material. They boxed her legs into broad, wide shapes in contrast to the shirt that clung needlessly to her waist and breasts. Yaniqui returned to the mirror to see the effect on herself. She looked like a slender shoot emerging from soft ground. She could get used to a life with poetry.

Yaniqui was hesitant to try the food ordering system, but her stomach demanded porridge and a nutrition packet. She pressed a button lightly near the dispenser. The cream cover of the dispenser sprang to life with pictures of different dishes. Yaniqui looked through the digital menu, selected her choice, and five minutes later, the cream cover slid open to reveal two dishes, a piping hot ceramic plate and a frosted glass bowl. She devoured the fruit quickly. She didn't even recognize the types, only knew anything that juicy and that sweet had to be grown on tall trees found on beautiful planets. Yaniqui ate the second dish of cubed, tender meat and fresh shoots much slower.

She wondered what Maemi thought of all of this. As someone more well-traveled than Yaniqui, Maemi wouldn't be so easily impressed, but she had to at least be pleased with the comfort and quality of everything around them. It beat living in the outer storage closet of a medical facility on 4,278.

Her doorbell rang, not that she needed to go and open it herself—in fact, she didn't have the key and couldn't leave—but it gave her a three-second warning to compose herself. She wiped her mouth, stood, and arranged the heavy trousers.

The attendant from last night stepped in. Her oval face was lit with a professional greeting.

"I'm to take you to the medical bay to make sure all is well." The woman's gaze traveled over Yaniqui's figure. "I see you've found the wardrobe. If there's anything you need, please let me know."

Yaniqui followed willingly but was uncomfortable that she didn't know what to call the woman and asked.

"Betha," she responded confidently. "And I already know yours, Yan-eh-key. You are to be a flower among petals." Betha smiled at Yaniqui as if she were sharing a secret, or perhaps a bit of good fortune.

Betha cued the door to open and they entered the wide hallway. Yaniqui enjoyed the way her slippered feet sank into the plush carpets. It wasn't hard to remember she had slept on a dirt floor until recently—it was more difficult to accept she wasn't dreaming everything in front of her. They stepped out of the quiet maze of halls filled with blank doors and into a much larger corridor. A man with a tray nodded respectfully to Yaniqui. He wore a cream smock identical to Betha's with a tiny crest of green in one corner. She couldn't help but smile back. At the juncture, Betha took a left and they exited onto a broad landing.

"You go first, I'll follow."

"Oh," Yaniqui said uncertainly, "I don't know where I'm going."

"Just to the bottom of the staircase. I'll follow behind and we'll make our way out together."

Yaniqui shrugged and started down. The moment her slipper lit upon the first step, the stairs turned golden in contrast to Yaniqui's dark pants while the elegant railings flashed the same fuchsia as her shirt. A laugh burst from Yaniqui and the few people below—some dressed in cream, others in a medley of different types of clothes—turned and beamed up toward Yaniqui.

By the third step, all felt right in the universe. Though Yaniqui was sure they were being polite, she had never seen a crowd look at her that way. She was more well-fed and comfortable than she could remember. It wasn't the path she expected to take, but she couldn't see why this one didn't end with an escape and Hloban after all. It was time fate gave her a break.

Betha and Yaniqui made their way through several more wide hallways—the spacecraft was absolutely huge—until they came to a light green door. Betha led her in, talked to the woman at the counter, and the three of them went back to a small private room. Betha peeked at a holographic screen while the other woman took Yaniqui's temperature and listened to her lungs.

Betha had just started a conversation about Yaniqui's curly hair when something pricked her inner arm. Startled, she automatically tried to pull away. The woman held tight to her forearm.

"Just taking a small sample." The woman didn't look up, but Yaniqui could see her cheeks lift in a neutral smile. "To make sure you're healthy."

When they finished, Yaniqui accepted a small square of gauze to wipe her arm clean but waved the bandage away. She didn't need to pretend. Betha was attentively watching, but it was the nurse whose attitude shifted to one of slight awe as the prick healed. The woman ran a finger across the place she had poked and looked at Yaniqui with an assessing frown.

Then Betha walked Yaniqui back while apologizing for the strenuous outing.

"No, it was quite fine."

"Well, I'm sure you'll want to rest either way."

Yaniqui was neatly deposited back in her room and she no sooner heard the door snap shut when it rang again. She turned, surprised Betha would return so quickly. Instead, a tall man stooped to enter her doorway and smiled. His crisp cream suit and dark green tie gave him a look of pure composure. A hint of cologne or aftershave filtered through the air.

"I apologize for calling on you so early in your day cycle, and before we've been formally introduced. My name is Hans Savini."

"It's very nice to meet you, Fra Savini."

His gaze ran up and down her body. "Fra Savini, how quaint. You can call me Mr. Savini."

Heat built in her cheeks and she looked at the man behind Hans Savini to distract herself.

Mr. Savini saw her attention shift. "Ah yes, the reason I've come unannounced. Karo, come in here."

A young man came in. His face was drained of blood as well as expression and he kept his eyes pointed at the floor. It was easy to see he was a worker but not on par with someone like Betha. He had a wide cream shirt covered with a pure white apron. The insignia for Akar stood out in green over one breast.

"Karo here," Mr. Savini's resonant voice spoke, "cut himself while cleaning the knives in the kitchen. Come here, Karo. Let's see what Yaniqui can do for you."

Yaniqui was taken aback. She hadn't expected to care for those on the ship, but it made sense as they were caring for her in their own ways as well. "Of course. Hold out your hand, please."

The cut on Karo's hand was deep, nearly to the bone. The familiar tang of iron fought against Mr. Savini's cologne to fill the air.

"Is it bad, miss? Will healing it hurt?"

Mr. Savini shot Karo a dark look and Yaniqui understood Karo's role was not to speak. This probably *was* the formal introduction. She only wondered if Mr. Savini waited until a member of the crew and staff got hurt, or if Karo was forced to injure himself.

"No, it won't hurt you at all. It will feel a little strange, and warm as your body goes to work, but I'll be doing most of it. My body provides the energy to your cells, but you will be very tired afterward." She wanted to calm Karo, but she said most of it for Mr. Savini's benefit. She supposed she'd have to get down a little routine if she was soon going to be healing high-class members. At least until she escaped.

The cut was easy to knit, and visual, exceedingly so that Mr. Savini filmed it with a device built right into his suit forearm. Yaniqui didn't notice until she was accepting Karo's thanks and shaking off the feeling of sliced meat.

Mr. Savini dismissed Karo.

"Well, that was something. I've been in the trade with Akar most of my life and have seen many different abilities at work, but seeing someone healed instantly…It's a shame you and your mother kept yourselves hidden away for so long. Think of all the good you could have done. Will do."

Yaniqui brushed her hands on her thick pant legs, trying to get the feel of Karo's clammy skin off her mind.

Mr. Savini snatched her wrist. "The blood, dear. Don't get it on the pants or we'll have to add it to your debt."

Indeed there was a smear of blood on Yaniqui's hand, but she was more focused on what Mr. Savini had said.

"Debt? How can I have debt if I'm currently owned by Akar Enterprises? I was told everything would be taken care of."

Mr. Savini bowed his head in regret. "Of course, my dear. It's not debt that you will ever have to worry yourself about but debt that will be billed to your new masters."

The relaxation, the luxury of it all, even the awkwardness with Karo, it all fled at the word *masters*.

Mr. Savini's arm beeped. He touched his pinkie and thumb together and the inside of his sleeve sprang to life with a screen that he read a notification on.

"Speak of the devil, and the devil shall appear with money in his hand. Or their hands in this case, Yaniqui. You have several interested buyers thanks to the confirmation of the blood work. And the video will further reassure them of your abilities."

A rush flew through her body. "Is that so?"

"Don't worry about a thing. We'll do an auction. We'll make all the arrangements. You relax"—Mr. Savini was heading to the door—"and we'll take care of the rest."

"But who are they? Who would want me?" She stumbled on the words.

"Cellular Researches for one. An old company, one we work with from time to time. They'd make you comfortable, I'm sure."

Yaniqui's voice lodged in her throat. Then it exploded. "You're going to sell me to a medical research company? They're not going to have me heal people—they're going to cut me open!"

Mr. Savini smiled kindly. "I doubt that. It'd be a terrible waste of their investment. But you should be pleased to know your mother was sold to a family, one who's represented on the Joint Council. That's very hush-hush of course, but they outbid a—"

"I want to see my mother." Maemi. She would make everything better. They could come up with a plan and fate would open the door to their escape. To Hloban.

Mr. Savini's brow wrinkled in an unnatural way. "That's not

possible, Yaniqui. Your mother's being prepped for departure now."

Yaniqui launched herself at Hans Savini intending to rake her fingers down his skin. He was prepared though and used her momentum to twist himself behind her. "Yaniqui, I can guess at what you're thinking. But I told you, I've been here for decades. There are two ways to do this. You can cooperate and live a good life, or you'll eventually be terminated, no matter how precious your abilities are. Service is better than that."

He spoke a voice command to the room and seconds later a guard appeared.

"Yes, sir?"

"Sedate the girl."

The guard took something from her belt. She put the small canister up to Yaniqui's arm and there was a click. Yaniqui howled, and moments later she was falling, further and further into herself, so far, she could finally see the truth.

She'd made a terrible mistake.

# Chapter 16
## Hloban
## In Transit

Yaniqui was in custody with Akar Enterprises—Hloban couldn't bring himself to use the phrase "owned by" as if thinking that was a crime in and of itself. The thought left him in a constant state of anxiety, anger ever near the surface. He was several hours into a deep search on the Interstellar Wave for information on where Akar held Yani. His eyes blurred and he blinked.

In the background, Waquas turned on the media dash for the Galaxy Championship Game of Routers and Adam sat down next to him on the squashy couch. Eeriva monitored the navigation and alert systems and Keyad slept. There was an unspoken rule that no one should interrupt Hloban while he researched. He didn't know if the others thought he was getting somewhere and didn't want to interrupt the lifesaving work, or if they knew he was reading and rereading the same articles and wanted to let him wallow in peace.

Either way, the sound of the game was on low for Hloban's benefit. He didn't look up until the audience cheer indicated halftime (the cheers during the matches were distinctly more divided in response).

"Strewth, look at that," Eeriva said loudly, Australian slang on display.

Hloban looked back and there was Yaniqui.

Indigo smoke rippled across the screen. She smiled one pure, jaw-dropping smile and Hloban's heart stopped. He would have known that curly black hair anywhere. She was no longer the skinny kid he went swimming with at Lake Venlu, or the lanky girl he exchanged gifts with on the New Year. She looked a little like Nica but didn't have the same straight nose. Hers was small and curvy. He wondered if she still had a light scar at the edge of her eyebrow. He'd forgotten about that scar until then.

Text rippled at the bottom of the screen, but Hloban missed it because someone dropped something. He looked down. It was him. He was shaking so hard he dropped a cup. By the time he looked back up, he got one more look at Yaniqui as she finished healing a woman's arm in demonstration before she was gone as quickly as she'd come.

"Was that her?" Adam asked, question hanging in the air while Hloban reassured himself he hadn't dreamed the whole thing up. A video clip of Yaniqui? During the Routers match? It was completely surreal.

"A commercial," Hloban said. He wasn't sure if he was asking or stating. "For Yaniqui?"

Hloban ran a hand over his face and felt someone touch his shoulder. He startled. It was Waquas. Well, now they knew what Akar was doing with Yaniqui. They were ready to sell. Already there had been photos and statements released as Akar built up awareness of one of their newest acquisitions. They were angling for a sale, maybe even an auction.

The room buzzed through the second quarter of the game as they discussed the advertisement and what it could mean. Eeriva was strangely silent, off-put by the whole thing. And Hloban didn't like how Adam kept exclaiming to his father, who had woken up from all the noise, "It was really her!"

"Uh, hey, guys. I think you're going to want to watch this," Waquas said.

Hloban refocused on the screen. It was another commercial break. A brief clip of a beautiful garden and outdoor tiled space in an elaborate estate panned past. Orange-capped mountains stood tall in the distance. Soft music played in the background. It was *that* kind of music. Hloban wanted to go back to the clinical advertisement of a product geared toward a medical research company or a government. Once he heard the music, he knew what other demographic Akar was targeting. They were selling an experience, one to those few beings out there that had the wealth to rival entire worlds. Want self-healing as part of your bloodline? You could have it.

A slip of a rumpled cover-up lay on the patio. A foot slowly came into view, a bronzed calf, and the thigh and the rest of…her, sleeping peacefully on an outdoor bed. Long arms and legs. Indigo Izbin silk hung overhead.

The screen went bright white and green text appeared: *Acquisition of a generation: Auction for Extreme Endangered Species from Wea Saa. Self-healing. The Ultimate Life-Enhancing Accessory.*

Hloban considered letting the auction play out. It would be easier to go up against one winning person or company, but there were too many unknowns. Yaniqui could be killed and dissected within hours of purchase. A warlord could impregnate her that day. She could disappear into thin air and reappear in another star system.

The only solid piece of information to focus on was that the sale would take place on Akar Evion, the big ones always did. But, as an invitation-only event, it was elusive as well. Jeb put Hloban in touch with a director of a human rights association, who apprehensively shared the location of Akar Evion with him.

"Every time the coordinates of Akar Evion are shared online, they're taken down within seconds," the director messaged Hloban. "Still, it's not that the location is a complete secret—there are too many workers and unfortunately too many clients—but I want to stress how well-guarded the planet is. I have enough to worry about without wondering if I sent an endangered species to his doom. But Jeb says you're smart enough, so please, *be smart enough.*"

Evion was one of twenty-five planets owned by Akar, a record number of planetary holdings for a nonagricultural corporation. Evion was not a casino, house of ill repute, playground for the rich, or any type of place one went to satisfy lusts, curiosity, or need. It was for processing. In their showrooms, one could buy any shape, age, size, or color of animoid or humanoid.

The Interstellar Wave had a few deep-net images of cells packed with animals or animoids and a few distant satellite images posted by an activist. Rumor had it that since the satellite images went public, there was a boom in new construction on the planet, including several sizable warehouses, perhaps for the sole purpose of making the earlier photos obsolete.

The more Hloban read about Akar, the more overwhelmed he was. He didn't know what Cortez was thinking. What he was thinking. It wasn't some basement operation that Hloban could set the police on or break up with a couple of semiautomatics.

Outright slavery was officially banned in the galaxy, but ownership was not. There was a subtle difference between the two that lobbyists and politicians fought fiercely over.

A slave was someone forcefully taken and held against their will. Petty kidnappings, child abductions, etcetera, etcetera. *Ownership* referred to legal holding of a being in pursuit of business and commercial interests. Someone could sign their life over to alleviate a debt or in exchange for food, shelter, and reasonable safety. Theoretically, a being could get out of debt or buy back ownership of themselves, but it almost never happened. Furthermore, in the underworld, the path to legal ownership of a person almost always started with an abduction. Then the captive was coerced or paperwork was otherwise falsified to create a clean trail. As long as the documentation said the right things, the being could be held as long as the owner desired and no one could contest it.

Manufacturing or sales of solid goods, even extremely valuable ones, could make you wealthy, but not as wealthy as Akar. Drugs were a close comparison. The same product could be sold to the same loyal customer base, an assurance of stable business. But the real key to extreme wealth, the sort the Akar empire had, was in selling the *same* resource over and over again. Akar was more similar to a landlord than a drug lord. A drug was used, gone forever except in the small molecules that became something else. However, a person sold for sex could be leased repeatedly in one day. A laborer could be signed out multiple times in a week. Even in the occurrence where ownership of the slave changed hands, there was a strong chance the being would come under Akar's charge again. Vulnerable people stayed vulnerable.

The business of ownership was a profitable one, but the more money corporations like Akar amassed, the more they had to buy out ambassadors or fund lobbyists or cover their tracks. Over time, Akar had built a layered web of vested interests of the wealthy and powerful, backed up by laws that said what they were doing was fair and reasonable.

One of the anxious thoughts that wouldn't leave Hloban alone was the question of how Yaniqui felt about all of it. At the start of the trip, Hloban had assumed Yaniqui would be happy to be rescued. That she'd risk her life to escape with Hloban. Out of loyalty to Loera, he tried to restrict his fantasies of rescue to the logistics of locating and saving Yaniqui. What mattered most was they would be reunited and Yaniqui would do everything she could to go with him.

Now he was not so sure.

Though he scoured the Wave, Hloban could not find a single fact or photograph of Yaniqui before her purchase. All he found were promotional items released by Akar. The same glossy photos of Yaniqui leaning toward a camera, her breasts nestled in lace. A video of Yaniqui demonstrating her healing abilities on herself and then on someone she called her best friend, a pink-haired woman also owned by Akar.

The thing that caught Hloban up most was how happy and natural she looked. She wasn't locked in chains. There were no dark circles under her eyes. She was well fed and when she laughed, her sharp incisors flashed.

The most damning thing of all was an official statement from Yaniqui, put out by Akar. In it, Yaniqui described how she attended university and earned high marks, but her mother passed away before she graduated. Hloban mourned the loss of Nica and knew Keyad was utterly devastated that the opportunity was lost to grow their Wea

Saavian colony on Earth by two. The statement went on to say that Yaniqui had big dreams and had carefully selected Akar to manage her career. She trusted them to make her a celebrity and find her a new home where she could use her gifts to better the galaxy.

Hloban reminded himself that that was how Akar worked. They wanted to make her story believable. They doctored information all the time. It was all promotional garbage Akar used to increase her value and make it seem like everything was done legally.

Though in his heart he knew that was the truth, he couldn't be totally sure. He didn't show the statement to Eeriva, terrified she would advocate for abandoning the mission. He might eject Eeriva if he heard her say that Yaniqui was better off, or ask who were they to interfere if that was what Yaniqui wanted. If it came down to it, he thought Cortez's office would back him up in hopes of becoming the famed home of the last female Wea Saavian, but he didn't care to test the waters.

Hloban had just read the official statement for the eighteenth time when he said, "I'm going to take the meeting with Onlo."

Keyad and Eeriva exchanged a glance.

Officially, the *Caneille* was on its way to Onlo, a corporation-owned planet specializing in technology across the spectrum. They created personal devices all the way up to large-scale resource management systems, like those for entire oceans. Both Onlo and most of Akar's land ownership were located in the same commerce hot spot. Hloban had set up the appointment with Onlo before they left the Orion Spiral Arm under the guise of discussing the sale of water. It gave them a final location to list on all immigration documentation, but the idea of meeting with Onlo was preposterous. Hloban didn't have any water holdings on planet Earth. As an alien, he wasn't allowed. Even Loera, as wealthy as her company was, didn't come close to the levels required for ownership of an ocean. And no one on Earth would ever ask *him* to broker a sale for them. Emmett wouldn't even give him fake documents before they left in the event that somehow it was all taken seriously and Hloban fucked up and sold the Pacific Ocean.

Still, Earth had copious amounts of salt water and was relatively unknown. The ambiguities fueled the corporations' interest in meeting him.

"To replenish our food, right?" Eeriva asked. "That's all, right?"

"Waquas," Hloban said, "Do we have enough time?"

Waquas pulled open the holo navigation and looked at it, then ran some calculations. He spoke without hesitation when he was finished. "Sure, but wouldn't it be better to be near Akar Evion in case we need to act early?"

"I think I can trade something to Onlo for supplies."

"Hloban," Keyad said slowly. "There's only one thing they would want from you besides water. What everyone else wants. Our blood."

"They don't just work in water security. They have weapons too. And we need food supplies."

Eeriva threw her hands up in the air. "I wanted to stop days ago and you bit my head off."

"It was always going to come to this," Hloban maintained. He saw the incredulous looks on everyone's faces. "This is my call to make."

Everyone was quiet over the next day as they made their way to Onlo. Besides the rare call to Earth and sending out routine paperwork to secure clearance to move through space territories, they had not been in contact with anyone. It felt strange to prepare to see someone entirely new after so many weeks cooped up in the *Caneille.*

When Onlo appeared within view, it glinted pale green. The shape clarified the closer they got and yellow shores and continents appeared along turquoise waters. At Onlo's checkpoint, Hloban insisted on disembarking by himself to the thermosphere station in a rented minicraft and then continue down to the planet surface on the space elevator. He reasoned that if something happened to him or he was delayed, the others could still get to Yaniqui in time.

He knew a break was also in order. Hloban suspected Eeriva talked about him back by the garbage receptacle to whoever would listen.

When Hloban came back from Onlo, he had a bandage on his arm, just as Keyad had said would happen.

Adam crinkled his nose in disbelief. "You did it? You gave them a blood sample?"

"I had to. But what I got in trade is much more valuable to us. Waquas, let's go."

Hloban waited until the planet was a tiny blip on their screen and then he pulled out his reward. He placed the heavy black box on the worn table. It looked and felt indestructible. Eeriva took in a sharp breath and Waquas stood up from the pilot's seat in shock.

"They gave you *that* for a vial of your blood?" Eeriva demanded.

"Let's try it out," Hloban said. He turned an intricate metal dial, nodded, and smiled.

"Nothing happened," Adam said.

Hloban laughed. He was actually going to save Yaniqui. He was going to do it. "You wouldn't know it, Adam, but we're invisible."

# Chapter 17
## Ippa
## In Transit

Dearest Bel,

I miss you and The Shou, of course, but I'm glad to have this opportunity to travel the galaxy. I'm currently on a large space transverser that includes me, the captain, eight crewmembers, and fifty-four laborers. We're all traveling to a remote planet where I plan to do original research.

I do feel much for the laborers. They're just hoping to find work and a planet untouched by war at the end of the journey, but you know what happens to refugees. Most likely than not, it ends badly. I've never been among the working class much. I have to admit, I miss the conversation of scholars.

**Ippa reread the last paragraph and deleted it. She wrote in its place:** It's so exciting being surrounded by different people. I'm learning a lot about other cultures.

My main duty on the transverser is to review the control system and look for snags within the framework. The captain called them bugs, but I don't know why he would assign the name of a group of beings to problems the original coders left behind.

When Ippa onboarded the collaborative craft, she was assigned to work in the kitchens, but she wasn't going to let any more opportunities pass her by. Ippa convinced the captain that she could deal with the coding issues. Ippa didn't tell him she wasn't a mainframe engineering student and the only interstellar flights she took were to and from Shou University. She also left out that she was currently banned from said university. But she could code well and made quick study of the transverser repair book, logs, and everything else she could read. Combing the system was a pleasant logical puzzle. Much easier than planning for the future.

The crew was surprised when I fixed the hot water in the rear W.C. Even the captain was impressed when I fixed an irregularity in the control panel display, though personally I'm alarmed that this crew has been traversing the galaxy while forced to multiply coordinates by 1.2 to find the correct placement of meteorites.

Life outside the scholarly life is a surprisingly restful experience. I feel like Long Tiraman when she went to live among the peasants and complete her work in quiet.

However, I am required to work out daily in the transverser gym to keep my muscle tone strong and, after a life of working with texts and data, it's a bit of a shock to the system! I'll be glad to get back to normal life when I arrive on-planet.

I'll be to my final destination soon, which I'm keeping secret for now.

**Ippa left out that she altogether decided not to notify her parents that she was traveling. In her mind, she justified the trip as a continuation of the education she started at the university, which they had agreed to let her attend. Her studies would simply be out in the field rather than in a classroom.**

Thanks for encouraging me and keeping in touch. I'll let you know how my research progresses.

Kisses and wishes,

Ippa

Ippa reread the message and sent it on to Bel. She had weird feelings about her friend who was still at The Shou (and therefore apparently better than her in every way), but Ippa hoped Bel would spread news about her adventure to their peers. And it was a true adventure, something she was convincing herself of more and more. Still, she had moments when she realized the date and felt the breathless thrill of upcoming finals, then realized she would never experience that side of life again.

Ippa walked to last meal and took her customary place next to the captain. He liked to hear about life at the university and tell tales of his voyages. Ippa saw members of the crew roll an eye on more than one occasion as he pontificated about the life of a leader.

"Can you tell me more about what the Jupiter Station is like?" Ippa asked. She tried to casually sprinkle in questions to their conversations to hide how ignorant she truly was regarding her travel plans.

"There's no need to worry," the captain said, mouth partly full of soy bread. "It's a small station, but it applies Joint Council regulation with all the fervor of that university of yours."

Ippa swallowed. The captain saw the panic on her face and waved a seven-fingered hand.

"Everything about the Station was designed for safety and immigration management. You will be fine, my dear. Though I will miss such cultured conversations. I hope we meet again on your way back out. It would be a pleasure to have you on my craft again. We traverse this route regularly."

Back in her bunk for her sleep cycle, Ippa shook. What was she doing way out at the far shores of civilization? Was it only because a professor assigned her Earth by chance for a research paper?

The thought that the Jupiter Station could turn her away for improper paperwork kept her awake. She didn't have the approval of The Shou, but she didn't think something like that would matter in a rural system. Parts of the planet didn't even have working lavatories, for crisp's sake! She expected her confident demeanor and the university's name, if not the credits, would be enough.

Ippa couldn't stand the thought of a second failure. More than that, she didn't have enough funds to go anywhere else. There was nothing left to do but move forward.

Ippa got out of the small bunk in her private, closet-like room and walked the hallways. The transverser was perpetually colder than Ippa was used to and she folded her arms across her chest to warm up. In the commons, she entered her account information to purchase a phone call. Ippa pushed away the desire to call her parents. Her mother could wait for the good news, whenever it arrived. Ippa dialed the last number she used to contact Earth. There was a heavy pause as the craft's technology tried to connect to a device on Earth. Ippa grabbed the roots of her blue hair and squeezed them in anxiety.

"Hello, Loera speaking." The voice sounded worried.

"Hi, Loera?"

"Yes. Yes, it is. Did something happen to Hoban?"

That name fired in her mind. It was the name of Loera's husband. "Oh, I don't think so. This is Ippa, the student who interviewed you about Earth."

"That's right. I remember you." Loera sounded instantly more relaxed. Ippa thought she could even hear Loera smile. "How did your project go?"

"Oh, well, my presentation was well-informed on current events thanks to you. I am, um"—Ippa had to steel herself to say it—"I am actually coming to Earth soon to gather samples and write a detailed report on the planet. Do you think we could meet in person?" Ippa held her breath, willing Loera to say yes.

"Wow, all the way to Earth? This must be some university. Of course, we can meet."

Ippa took a deep breath and her shoulders relaxed. She even smiled.

"Do you have a place to stay?" Loera asked. "We'd love to host you at our home. My schedule's pretty busy with work, but we have a lot of friends in the expat community who would enjoy talking with you. You could come see my lab, if you like," Loera said the last bit a little shyly for her outgoing personality.

Ippa didn't expect it to be so easy. "Yes. Thank you. I'd love to stay at your home." Ippa took a breath and tried to control her excitement. "Staying in an Earth home would be a great cross-cultural experience."

"This is good timing because we have another guest coming soon.

My husband is on a retrieval voyage right now. I can't tell you everything over the connection, but he's helping a young girl from his old home planet immigrate here. They're both of an extremely endangered species. She was being trafficked, if you can believe that. Having someone else from off-planet might ease her transition into life on Earth."

Ippa's mind spun at the thought of meeting someone who was trafficked. It was a bit more real-world than anything she ever thought she'd engage with in the real world.

"I'd love to meet them both. I'm on my way to the Jupiter Station now. I'll get in touch when I'm closer to Earth. Thanks again, Loera."

"Safe voyage."

Ippa hung up the receiver and whooped. She was so excited that she ran down the corridor in her pajamas. She heard the captain's voice call down the hall, "That's the way to apply yourself, Ippa. Let's bring that motivation to the gym."

The next morning, Ippa packed up her two bags, returned books to the tiny onboard library, and finished a last bit of code she wanted to get in as thanks for a successful voyage. There was a constant buzz of energy in the halls as people readied themselves for transition.

Ippa peeped out a porthole. The Jupiter Station was small. Or was it that the planet was so big? White, orange, and red swirled across the surface of the gas giant. A thrill of exhilaration turned in her stomach. This was it. Her big adventure. She was going to make the most of the experience.

She'd be on the Jupiter Station for two rotations around the planet while they looked over her paperwork and watched for any signs of physical illness. The Earth population had little immunity to the varied diseases that roamed the galaxy from one unwashed hand to another and took communicable sicknesses seriously.

If all went according to plan, Ippa wouldn't pay anything. Whereas she knew from conversations with the captain that the laborers received a migratory discount but would still owe a hefty debt by the time they arrived on-planet. They'd have to work to pay that back as well as settle their families. Earth offered short-term deferred loans followed by large interest rates.

However, an educational and cross-cultural exchange would permit her free entry to Earth for a limited time. The Educative Experience Program, a student exchange, worked on a quid pro quo basis. Earth last utilized the program three standard years prior and they were probably eager to have a visitor so that they could send out another Earthling on a research mission.

She figured strings would be pulled in her honor just so Earth could continue participating in the program. Word would travel ahead of her. She wouldn't be surprised if meetings and tours were arranged and in place by the time she arrived on-planet.

*Vrrrmmmmm*

"Please wait."

*Vrrrmmmmm*

"Just a little more."

*Vrrrmmmmm*

"There. That will do it." Ippa locked gazes with the technician, an Earthling male.

Men and women from Ippa's home planet were typically of a height. Balanced chores and equal nutrition paid off for everyone. But Ippa read about this phenomenon in her research. Men were generally taller than women on Earth, sometimes significantly so. With a large sample of Earthlings in front of her, she could see that, yes, weirdly enough, the women were shorter as a rule. Except she shouldn't think of it as weird. That was Ren Persimm's second rule of astro anthropology. To never think of things in terms of normal or abnormal. Rule one was to never eat or drink something that clashed with your molecular microbiology just for the sake of your anthropological work.

Still, Ippa was a little disappointed the tech was her height. She always pictured Earthling males as huge and strange.

He looked up, and shook back his auburn hair to better smile at her. Well, Ippa considered, this way was good too.

He started the encounter with a scripted explanation of her rights and which rights she forfeited by traveling into the Sol System, one of which was a complete inspection of her belongings. Another tech would inspect her body. He blushed at that part of the explanation.

"How long have you lived on the Jupiter Station?" Ippa asked. She knew her accent would sound different to him.

"Almost two Earth years. Not that that means much out here." He flipped through her items by hand now that he was sure there were no dangerous powders, spores, or insects. "Long enough to get used to it, I guess."

"And you were a child when the station was constructed?" Ippa asked.

"No, maybe when my parents were children. I've always known about the station and the existence of others. Contact and all, you know. My parents had a hard time with it though."

"And now you are working out here. Is that hard for them?" Ippa asked.

"My mama's passed, but it is hard for my dad. He thinks it's unsafe and not a very good job. He wishes I worked in coastal restoration like him."

*Oh my.* The Earthling pulled her underwrap out of her bag, but he didn't seem to know what it was. He flipped it around and looked at it carefully. Ippa's nipples burned. She had only two with her. One was tucked around her breasts right now. In an instant, she knew she wouldn't wash it before wearing it again, even if she had the chance.

He moved through the rest of her bag deftly. He paged through her books and ran a translator glass over a few random passages. Satisfied they were educational materials, he picked up another, smaller book and looked at the cover. There, on the front, was an illustration of two different species of animoids locked in a moist embrace.

She saw the man's mouth curve at the edges.

"That's not mine," Ippa blurted.

The man's expression went from sly to shock. "Ma'am, did you pack your bag? Did someone place an unknown object in your bag?"

"No-no, that's not what—"

*"Code four!"* he bellowed.

Ippa heard a thunderous click as doors locked seconds later. Half the people in the room got on the ground and sheltered under tables.

The other half converged on Ippa.

"I borrowed it from the spacecraft library and didn't give it back!" Ippa said in a rush. "That's what I meant when I said it wasn't mine."

A supervisor who appeared at the tech's elbow scrunched her eyebrows. "I assume you'd rather keep this piece of literature than pay to reopen the bay and return it?"

Ippa meekly nodded her assent and the supervisor leaned against the table to watch the rest of the proceedings. The red-faced tech checked through the rest of her supplies, this time avoiding Ippa's eyes.

# Chapter 18

Lozen
The Catchment, Earth

Lozen walked back to the Catchment. She wasn't tired, but her bag was full enough with asparagus, morels, and bunches of fresh greens like ramps and chickweed. Very early spring was a cold time of year for foraging and Lozen was grateful for what she found. Windburn licked her cheeks and her lips were chapped, but she didn't mind. Her skin was usually roughed with something or other. True solitude, the type she could find outside the muddy and ever-reeking scent of packed bodies in the Catchment was rare and worth the trade of comfort.

Ever since Lozen navigated the dark caves and appeared before the Karmas, her initiation was on her mind. Charla clearly expected her to figure out how to identify and locate a terrorist, then bring him to justice, whatever that meant. Lozen did look. Randomly and sporadically but enough to demonstrate to the Karmas that she was making an effort. But the more time passed, the less likely it seemed that Lozen was going to solve the case and be accepted into the family of the Karmas.

It was clear enough to Lozen when the Catchment was close. Dead trees stripped of bark stood crooked in the ground. It was muddy from children playing in the snowmelt. She put her foodstuffs inside her sweatshirt and made her way to her one-room house. Mama Teresa sprawled in the doorway of her haphazardly leaning shack. Now that it was warm, or at least warmer, Mama Teresa abandoned the purple handout coat like everyone else. She wore the same patterned red sweater every day, matted and oily along the left sleeve.

Lozen ignored Mama Teresa and went inside her own house. She put half of the supplies she gathered in a canister, buried it, and packed the dirt down hard. Lozen kicked loose dust over it and replaced the fabric she used as a rug. She fingered the slightly prickly line underneath her hair and uncomfortably thought about her next move.

She split the rest of the foraged food between two bags and walked immediately next door. She knew the lives and fights and fart jokes of the family of eight that lived there, better than even herself. After all, she never talked to herself and all she had to listen to were those around her.

"Marcie, *tep tep*?" Lozen said outside the open door.

"*Tep.*" The mother of the bunch nodded her way, her hands full of baby. Lozen didn't see Jerramy so she gave Uzzie the plastic bag. "Bring this to your mother, Uzzie." Uzzie opened it to look and a little one darted in, took a morel, and licked it, dirt and all. Lozen swiped it back in the bag, and gave Uzzie a push toward his mom.

Marcie had her shirt pulled up because she was breastfeeding, and Lozen couldn't help but see her stomach. It was puffy from Marcie's most recent pregnancy except around the belly button that wrinkled dramatically, as if to express its displeasure at no long being stretched to popping.

Marcie and Lozen exchanged a few sentences, but Lozen could tell Marcie was barely present. She was exhausted by the sheer act of keeping her family alive with the addition of the new one. It wore on Lozen too. She woke in the night every time the baby cried and struggled to get back to sleep in the cold. Sometimes she did knee-lifts to warm herself until the baby quieted. Lozen would be warmer if she shared a house with someone, but without her aunt, Lozen couldn't imagine who that someone would be.

Lozen left and walked down the dirty path, reviewing her plan on the way. She had gone into the forest for a reason. After weeks of no headway on finding the bomber, and no subsequent attacks, Lozen had little faith she was going to discover anything at all. She didn't want to embarrass herself, of course, but the real pang came when she thought about losing the chance to be a part of a group of women who seemed like a family, one she didn't want to admit to herself how desperate she wanted to be a part of.

Lozen rounded the corner to the bombing site. Ahead were six Catchment regulators plus a man and a woman in formal clothing. They were talking to an older local who spoke heatedly and pointed his finger in their faces before walking away. He turned to glare at the officers once before fading into a small group of residents.

Lozen scratched her neck while she watched the unfamiliar woman and man. They both had shimmering badges on their shoulders. Lozen was struck dumb for a moment. They were holos. Badge numbers floated over the top of the smooth metal. Regulators had already been out to the site several times. These were outside government officials.

Lozen slid over to an elder with a sunken mouth.

"Have those people been here long?"

The woman shrugged. "They been here lookin' around, scraping the ground, talking to everybody. Everybody but me it seems. They talked to her." The woman pointed across the ruins. "Why don't you go ask her?"

"I thought you'd know."

The woman yelled across the way to the other in another language. "She said they were ge ai aye."

"GIA?"

"S'what I said." The woman was done with Lozen and walked away.

Lozen wrinkled her nose. Now she understood why the old man was so upset. Though the Catchment started as a place for HUD to crowd in the homeless they didn't want to deal with, it later came under GIA jurisdiction when the government began moving newly arrived alien refugees in. The GIA department came into the Catchment every once in a while and nearly always left it worse off. They arrested young men and women for trying to make money to support their families. Lozen didn't care what someone decided to do, whether it was sell drugs like perval or their bodies. If it kept food in kids' bellies, it was necessary. The GIA felt differently. And when they took breadwinners away, it left families more vulnerable than before.

Lozen stayed until the outsider group left in two pristine black trucks. A young man spit after them and hurried away, as if escaping immediate confrontation.

At the blackened building, Lozen looked at what was left. The acrid smell of soot mingled with charred wood and the sour scent of melted plastic. Footing was hard to keep among the rubble. Lozen wasn't the only one in the bomb site. As soon as the strangers left, people converged as they had ever since the site stopped smoldering. Two men stacked bricks on a piece of tin to carry away. A pack of dirty kids, one of whom had snot running down his upper lip, climbed on big pieces of fallen ceiling. The booger boy licked his lips.

The wood of the building was long gone, but Lozen worked at clearing stones from the station's back room and hoped something would occur to her as to the motives of the bomber or his identity. Nothing did.

She didn't want to do what she had planned next, but it was the only avenue left.

She jumped down from a small broken hunk of concrete.

"Hey, what's wrong with your mouth?" booger boy said and stared.

"Fuck off."

Lozen walked away quickly but still heard the shocked laugh of a kid behind her. She slowed once she was out of sight.

She was far away when the quality of Catchment homes shifted. These were the blocks HUD originally built to rehabilitate the homeless. The two hundred original shelters. They were fancy with proper concrete walls, floors, and shingled roofs. Even pit latrines. The pit latrines were long since filled with debris and many of them were buried over, but these blocks remained the envy of everyone else.

At one house, there was an unusual crowd and a line of people outside the door. That was it, Lozen was sure. She took a place and squatted with her back to the concrete wall.

*What's wrong with your mouth?*
*I ate too many boogers.*
Yeah, that's what she should have said.

Lozen spent the better part of the afternoon waiting and listening to small conversations. When a stout-looking woman finally beckoned Lozen in, she stood and stretched. Inside, a young man frisked her and searched her bag before giving it back.

She was shown to a low table. Opposite her was a man with so many fine wrinkles, he looked like a lined leaf. In contrast to the delicate skin, a bulbous nose sat squarely in the middle of his face. He bid her to sit. Fire burned in a metal container and Lozen flexed her hands, eager for the warmth.

"I've not seen you before," Lin said. "I would remember your split lip."

Lozen ignored the comment and took three bundles of asparagus out of her bag, using the opportunity to compose her face while she looked down. "I found these in the woods."

Lin laughed in surprise. "My parents used to collect asparagus. So, you are one of those that walks far, huh? Me, I haven't been past the fence in years. Everything I need is in this house."

Lozen smiled and looked around the room politely. "They're tender. And they're for you."

Lin nodded at the woman who stood in the doorway and she took the asparagus away. Lozen watched the food disappear a little sadly.

The resources secured, Lin was ready for business. "Now, what would you like? If you're after a cut of preval, you will need to give me more than that. If you're after a husband, you'll need a lot more. I'll have trouble finding someone who will take you with that damaged lip. Though"—he looked Lozen up and down—"not bad otherwise. Let me see your teeth."

"No, no," Lozen said hastily. "I'm here because I was there when the handout station went up in smoke. Everyone's been saying, well, that the person who did it is still out there. I want to help out any way I can."

Lin reached across the table for her hand. "A young one like you shouldn't worry. Of course, we are all concerned. You must be scared, hmm?" He stroked her hand and wrist.

Lozen forced herself to look him in the eye as she pulled back. "I can keep an eye out for things if I knew what to look for."

Lin wrinkled his face even more. He sat back and straightened. "Why's a woman like you want to get mixed up in men's affairs for?" He angled his body away, toward the fire, and halfheartedly threw a hand up. "It's dinnertime. You need to go back to your family. We'll handle this."

Lozen didn't give her food away to leave with nothing. She bit her anger down. If he wanted a demure woman, that's what he'd get. "I'm just—just so upset." She hunched her shoulders as if she were about to cry.

Lin patted Lozen's hands more platonically this time. "Everyone wants to know who did it, but you don't need to worry about it. Bring me more asparagus if you find some." He put his hand below the table and started scratching. "You want some preval? I'll give you a discount for your first time. Take it with a friend."

"It's—" Lozen continued, determined to keep Lin on track. She let her voice catch, more natural than she expected. "It was terrible. My dad has been upset ever since. He said he heard the GIA was here today."

"You tell your father the GIA won't be back. They're just making show. This will all be handled here in the Catchment. I already have reports from the south quadrant." Lin stood. "You send your dad to me when you're ready for a husband."

"Thank you for keeping the Catchment safe." Lozen smiled, before leaving.

The next morning, Lozen hit up the small market in the south quadrant. It wasn't a forbidden market by any means. It was the U.S. government's greatest dream that the Catchment would be able to feed and trade among themselves and allow the rest of the world to forget about them.

Lozen traded some of her watercress for three strips of jerky from Madame Asnel and ate two crouched by a pile of garbage as she watched. Nothing happened. It was a waste of a morning and her teeth hurt from the hard meat.

The sky was heavy with gray clouds and Lozen smelled fresh musk. She hurried to get home before the clouds broke.

There was nothing left to do but tell the Karmas she couldn't do it. Lozen played out several scenarios in her head, each one more embarrassing than the last, with Charla's face always a beautiful sneer. It would be better to cut things off as soon as she could.

Lozen's tin door was slightly out of place. She peered in and laughed.

"How's it, sister?" Monte lay on Lozen's pallet, chewing gum, with her legs up against the wall.

Monte sat up. They slapped hands and Lozen joined her friend. Monte ran her fingers through Lozen's hair, finding the shaved portion and scratching playfully, then rested her head on Lozen's shoulder. "I stopped by earlier today too, but you weren't here."

"I went to the market to trade some foods and Madam Asnel had some not-too-old jerky. Her goat died."

"And you wanted a bite of that dirty old thing? He was such an asshole."

"Which made him all the more delicious." In reality, it was difficult eating. Two of Lozen's back teeth pained her and one was definitely loose. She figured she had to get them pulled but worried that was the catalyst for becoming one of the old, weathered grandmothers along the lane.

They switched to whispers.

"Monte, I'm going to tell the Karmas I can't do it."

"Sure you can," Monte said. "They know you can. They wouldn't have accepted you just because you're my friend."

"Why's it all so secret?"

Monte thought. "Honestly, I think they're tired of being laughed at by their husbands and boyfriends. Once you're initiated, I'll tell you all about the stuff they're doing to taunt Lin's gang."

Rain broke with a thunder of raindrops on Lozen's tin roof. It was likely only a drizzle. The tin made everything more dramatic than it actually was.

They sat quietly for a moment. Monte spun a rope bracelet on her wrist. "I wasn't able to tell you about my initiation before," her words faltered, "but I had to find a girl who went missing. Her name was Lilly."

Lozen's heart sank at the past tense. "What did you do?" Lozen asked.

"Probably what you're doing right now. I wandered randomly. I hung around a few brothels and I checked the quarry for her body. I told a few washerwomen I was looking for my sister, but no one saw Lilly. There was only one place left to go: the animoid blocks."

A drop of wet fell on her hand. She put her arm around Monte.

Monte's voice rasped as she tried to keep quiet while crying. "When anyone wants to join the Karmas, they think they're going to be a hero, but everyone else's initiation story is as pathetic as mine." Monte took a deep breath. "Lilly had been gone for several days at that point. If she was alive, someone would have brought her home. So, I…" Monte paused, unsure what her oldest friend would think. "I asked to buy body parts."

Lozen looked at her friend's face in the dim light, shocked.

"I know, it makes me sound like a monster to even think of it."

"No," Lozen started to say, but Monte kept talking.

"There was this underground store, literally underground. Lozen, I hardly believed it. There were human bodies. On one rack was the skinned body of a child, with a little red hair still on the scalp. Lilly had red hair. I was furious. There was this disgusting nonperson there, one of them with a beak mouth. I saw a gas canister, took a lighter out of my pocket, and turned it on. I told the ugly thing I was taking the body, or we could both burn to death. I was serious. I would have burned before I let someone eat or magic Lilly." Monte's face crumpled even more and she brought her hands up to cover her mouth. "Bringing Lilly's body back to her parents was the hardest thing I've ever done."

"Monte, I'm so sorry." Lozen wiped her own tears away. "Why

bother with the Karmas? If they made you do that?"

"Don't you see, Lozen? They're the only ones trying to protect people. The initiation is there for a reason. You get stronger." Monte stood up and wiped her eyes on her sleeve. "I have to get back. Gabby hasn't been well and my mother will need me to sit up with her. I just wanted to check on you."

They hugged good-night and Monte left.

Lozen sat for a little while. When the rain showed no signs of stopping, she peed in a basin and chewed a peeled twig, tentatively tapping her back teeth and wincing when they predictably hurt.

She kept imagining her sweet friend surrounded by the meat of humans.

She finally laid down when the rain went quiet. She dozed and rolled and felt a hand cover her mouth. An iron forearm pinned her shoulders. Lozen felt for the handle of a rusty scrap under her mat and shoved it with all of her force into the person's abdomen.

Instead of sticking in and running hot blood, the blade deflected and fell to the dirt floor. She lost her grip on it and thrashed, trying to pick it back up. The person hissed and struggled with Lozen to keep her still. Lozen felt herself lifted off the mat as if she were a child and thrown on her stomach. A body sat on her back and pulled up an arm at a sharp angle.

A whisper came to her ear, "GIA. Remain calm and I'll let you up." Though the woman hissed her words, her accent was television-ready, prim and clipped.

"Do you understand? Nod."

Lozen nodded and the woman tentatively lifted her hand. Assured that Lozen wasn't going to scream, she took it away entirely but kept her weight on Lozen's back a few seconds more. Then she got up and waited for Lozen to lift herself off the ground.

"We can't talk here, but I have a job for you."

Lozen couldn't see her but wondered if it was the woman from the bombing site the previous day.

"I'm not interested. Get out of here," Lozen said. She didn't want to think about what would happen if she was caught working with law enforcement.

"You'll be interested when you hear what you'll get in payment. You don't want to live in this shack forever." The voice sounded as if it was generously offering a great gift.

Lozen breathed deeply and whispered back, "No, you don't understand. I'll be crucified if anyone in the Catchment finds out I even talked to you."

The woman thrust something into Lozen's hands. It felt heavy and expensive. "Meet me at dawn in the forest at these coordinates. Make sure you're not followed and don't tell anyone." She disappeared behind the hanging blanket.

Lozen shook, the adrenaline from the encounter disappearing as rapidly as it had come. She wondered if she was going to be sick. After a moment, she stood and replaced the thick tin door. She wasn't sure what had felt worse, the moment she was sure she was going to be robbed or when the woman said *GIA*.

Galactic Intelligence Agency.

# Chapter 19
## Hloban
## Akar Evion

Keyad, Adam, and Hloban, three of the last five known Wea Saavians, leaned against the tiny spacecraft windows while Waquas and Eeriva manned the console as they landed on Akar Evion. The planet was small as far as planets went, but there was still plenty of space for Akar to expand. The main compounds were surrounded by large swaths of empty grasslands, probably to purposefully exempt any natural features that could aid a slave to escape undercover.

After weeks of navigating remotely and running on autopilot most of the time, Waquas finally had a chance to actually pilot the *Caneille*. Invisible and purposefully avoiding communications with the navigation tower, it was difficult to know where to land. They finally decided to alight near a large compound they believed was holding facility 12A based on the research and satellite photos Hloban had accumulated.

Though Hloban knew the cloaking device from Onlo was infallible, he still expected guards to rush them the moment the landing gear touched ground.

Nothing happened. Which also made Hloban nervous.

"Oh fuck," he said. "If we're invisible, could someone see the bent grass where we landed?"

Adam lurched up to look out a porthole but that wouldn't tell them anything.

Eeriva shook her head. "There's no one here, we're a quarter mile from the compound."

In the end, Hloban made Waquas move to "that patch of dirt over there" and then Adam saw a dirt patch that looked less grassy than the one Hloban had found. Waquas assured them that though security was terribly good, nobody in the crisping universe had time to examine individual blades of grass.

Hloban wore a thick jacket with the purpose of stowing a small handgun inside, two OxLit devices, and a Wipeout Con, all of which he had said nothing about to the others, not even when he initially bought them on Onlo.

He kept patting his jacket where the Con was stored, nerves shooting whenever it occurred to him that he hadn't checked it recently. The Wipeout Con was a self-guiding dart with immense breakthrough power that, when it hit its target, would suck oxygen out of the air within seconds. Hloban didn't plan to set off the molecular reaction unless he had to. It was a deadly decision and more than once, he wished he hadn't taken it from Onlo, but how else could he walk inside Akar without the type of weapon that would give them pause if he was cornered?

If he was forced to set it off during their escape, the OxLits in his jacket were to supply him and Yaniqui with oxygen. The reaction would ravage an enclosed space instantaneously. If he activated the Con in 12A, nearly all the staff and captives would die. But those lives were already forfeit. Hloban would prefer to die quickly than be used for labor and testing the rest of his life, but he knew Waquas would disagree.

The auction was scheduled to take place that evening and Yaniqui was surely on Akar Evion already. The others had fought Hloban when he said he would go in alone. He responded that one person would be more inconspicuous, but in his heart he knew that he had to save

Yaniqui by himself. He didn't have much of a plan—find her, release her, bring her back to the ship—but he did believe in his ability to do what needed to be done as it came. Maybe he was married to Loera now, but he still had an unbreakable bond with Yaniqui. The stars determined they be together. Somehow, it was going to happen. He would save Yaniqui.

Hloban shook hands with Keyad and hugged Adam. Waquas nodded at him and Eeriva grasped him hard by the shoulders and peered into his eyes, checking for his sanity probably. Loera and Obani came to his mind and his chest seized up at the thought of never seeing them again. But it inflated when he thought of seeing Yaniqui. Very soon.

A siren wailed across the compound. Everyone peered at the screen or out one of the few portholes, but there was no immediate change to the blue sky, grassy expanses, or industrial center.

"What is that?" Adam asked. "Do they know we're here?"

Waquas listened carefully. "Something escaped. They're locking down the planet."

"How do you know that?" Adam asked.

Hloban started for the door of the craft. "I'm going, then. I have to go now."

Eeriva pulled back on his arm. "Wait, Hloban, let's at least figure out what escaped. You're going to want to stay away from that area. If you go now, we can't communicate once you leave the range of the cloaking device."

Hloban had decided not to bring a communicator of any type with him. It was sure to be picked up by the planet surveillance system.

Something drove fast down a black industrial road below them. Without being asked, Waquas manipulated the screen and brought up a closer image. It was a half-capsule hovercraft, the sort used in manufacturing facilities, just big enough to move one person to the other side of a work site quickly. The top was open. A uniformed guard wearing a helmet was driving.

Akar-marked crafts took to the air now. Were they doing sweeps of the ground? What went missing? This nonsense was going to delay him. Hloban's heart sped at the thought of coming this close and missing Yaniqui.

The hovercraft stopped in front of a warehouse of some kind. Hloban had seen it on the satellite photos as well. It was a heavy titanium structure.

The person had trouble stopping the hovercraft and spilled out of the capsule, fell on the ground, and struggled to rise in a too-big uniform. Once on his feet, he made his way to the main door and slid up the visor of his helmet.

Hloban gripped the navigation chair in front of him tightly and Waquas turned back in confusion, but Hloban's eyes were on the screen. It wasn't a guard. Her hair was black.

"That's Yaniqui!"

Eeriva already had a holo open in front of her, marking out a path in 3-D with her hands. "I'm sending out one of our drones. Maybe it will get ignored in all the confusion. We need a higher view on this to see what's going on and where she goes."

"Why is she going in there? Come this way," Adam shouted as if Yaniqui could hear his advice.

At the door, Yaniqui's borrowed uniform fell and revealed a thick black space jumpsuit.

"There must be spacecrafts inside. She's going to try to run for it," Hloban said.

Yaniqui pulled out a card, scanned it, and typed in an additional code. Even from that distance, Hloban could see her hands shake while he froze with indecision. He could jump from the *Caneille* and give her away or see what plan she had and be too late.

"Let's at least get off the ground and move closer. Waquas, do you think you can fly low enough to not get in the way of the Akar crafts?"

"We can try, but we can't get too close to the compound without giving ourselves away. They can still hear our engine."

Light shone brilliantly off the polished door as it rolled open on its track.

From the open mouth of the warehouse, dark and twisted smoke poured out. Darker and denser than any smoke Hloban dared imagine. It wrapped around Yaniqui, nearly enveloping her. She put a hand in front of her face as if she could shield herself, straightened her shoulders, and walked in.

"What the hell—" Eeriva said.

Hloban froze and made eye contact with Keyad as the realization sprang upon them. He saw his horror and disbelief reflected back. Hloban's head was going to burst. "What the fuck are they doing with that? What is she thinking?"

In the distance, a private craft lit to life in the sky park. A set of uniformed guards with rifles raised converged on the ship, stopping it from flying away. Another ship lit up seconds later and the guards split in half to keep both crafts grounded. They signaled at those in the craft to open their doors.

"We need to get out of here," Eeriva directed. "This mission is over."

Yaniqui was gone from view, lost in the tendrils of smoke.

Four large vehicles pulled up to the warehouse but not nearly as close as Yaniqui's discarded hovercraft. Guards on foot approached, but no one went in. Hloban could imagine their apprehension. His soul mate was over there, and he didn't want to approach either.

Grief washed over Hloban. He had been so close to her. He didn't know how she could have escaped or possibly have gotten ahead of her captors, but she must not have known what she would find in the warehouse.

A bracing roar screamed its way across the grass plains of Akar Evion.

The hairs on Hloban's neck stood and he imagined every being alive turning its head to the cry in meek fear. The echoing scream was the timeless sound of death and destruction. It was evolutionarily hardwired into Hloban's brain to flee anything that powerful, that berserk.

The barren planet sprang into action. More crafts lifted into the air from several different lots. A civilian took off despite the frantic waves of a ground marshal.

An Akar jet targeted a fleeing craft and two puncture marks showed on the side of the private vessel. It spun twice, gained control, and made a heavy landing on the ground.

Keyad and Eeriva set controls as fast as they could alongside Waquas to take them up into the upper atmosphere.

"What are you doing? No, no, we're going to get her." Hloban threw himself over Keyad's arm and flipped off switches. He couldn't let them leave without Yaniqui.

Eeriva hit him hard in the chest with her elbow and pushed him out of the way. "Adam, hold him down."

"Listen, Hloban," Adam said. He looked like a boy. "I have no fucking idea what's happening, but stay away from the controls and we won't have a problem." A scared boy.

Hloban barred his teeth at Adam's outstretched hands.

The *Caneille* buzzed to life and jarred off the ground. Something dark poured out of the warehouse. Fluid and seamless black smoke rippled through the air. The crew stared, eyes wide, feud forgotten. Within the clouds of haze was a beast, twisting and turning, unraveling snakelike onto the ground of the planet. One of the vehicles aimed to attack with a top-mounted cannister. The monstrous beast lashed out and the security vehicle bent and melted.

Enormous titanium bands stretched across the colossal reptile's frame but hung loose and unlocked. It shook its head and thrashed its tail against the warehouse, which quivered upon impact.

Space cruisers continued to blast off the planet surface while a group of fighter jets flew in formation straight toward the dragon. One craft swerved away, its pilot deciding to save his own life.

"I don't believe it," Keyad said. He pointed his finger right up against the screen.

Hloban squinted. There! On the back, obscured partly by the wings of the beast, was Yaniqui.

Hloban dived at the controls again. "We can't leave her! Gods, she's going to burn."

Eeriva pulled on Hloban with all her might. "We can't help her. We need to leave *now*. I've seen pictures of the remains of planets when those things are mad, and that one has been caged by an interstellar slaver and it is pissed! Fly Waquas or so help me *gods!*"

The ship suddenly bolted in the opposite direction of the dragon. Eeriva and Hloban fell solidly to the floor. Eeriva's hip landed on

Hloban's knee and he groaned even as she rolled off.

The rear cameras showed an explosion that punctured the air behind them. A great cloud of fire leaped into the sky. Seconds later, a wave of tension rocked the *Caneille* in a heavy wash of wind that made the metal and steel creak.

"Shit," Adam whispered. "Waquas, go faster," he said, eyes wide.

Keyad redirected the rear cameras to track the dragon. He jerked unconsciously when he saw the animoid switch direction midflight like a snake striking. It landed briefly on the ground to barrage a rolling vehicle with heavy artillery attached to the side. A massive tail struck one side of the tank as Hloban thought of it. It crumpled upon impact. The dragon moved on, screaming as it flew low across the ground, its mouth open. Behind it, vehicles melted and burst into flame.

"Dad, what is that?" Adam sounded terrified. Hloban felt the same.

"It's a dragon." Keyad's clammy skin had taken on a sheen of sweat. "Dragon fire only spreads."

"She's dead. She's got to be dead."

"Shut up," Hloban bellowed.

The animoid flew faster than any vessel Hloban had ever seen and with more fluidity than any robotic counterpart could. The creature snapped around to take a low-flying craft out of the sky with its jaws. The dragon launched higher into the sky, setting one ship ablaze and sent it spiraling to the ground.

*We're invisible, we're invisible,* Hloban repeated to himself. The dragon pounced and relaunched off an escaping craft. To his horror, the dragon pulled even with the *Caneille.* Eeriva put a hand over her mouth and Keyad pulled his son in close.

The dragon was so close the craft shuddered from the sheer velocity of the creature. Spikes lined the dragon's back and face except for a mass of off-color gray scars on the neck. Hloban wanted to close his eyes but couldn't.

A small, endlessly silver eye flitted over to the invisible, untraceable spacecraft and rested there.

The dragon ceased to be muscle and armor and became energy, an endless energy of flame and destruction, defense and fight. It was a boiling mass of power and sprang at the *Caneille*.

A fighter jet dived under the beast to escape and instead collided with the dragon. In the moment before the blast, there was Yaniqui. Hloban couldn't see her face—the helmet was sealed and her head was buried in her lap. That she could hold on, that she could withstand the heat and force was impossible. It was utterly incomprehensible, but nothing made sense.

Hloban was going to die. They all were. It was his last chance to tell Yaniqui he had come for her. With shaky hands, he queued up the speaker control when Eeriva and Keyad tackled him.

"Are you trying to bring that thing down on us?" Eeriva hissed as they pinned Hloban to the floor.

The dragon leaped over the *Caneille*, disappearing from the screen and porthole windows.

Everyone held their breath. Waquas frantically redirected the cameras and they saw the dragon—and Yaniqui—flying up into the atmosphere, away from them.

# Chapter 20
## Yaniqui
## Akar Evion

Wind ripped at Yaniqui's jumpsuit. It tore at her gloved hands as if it were alive, desperate to consume her. Yaniqui's eyes watered under her helmet visor. Even if she could have rubbed them she never could have loosened one hand from the scaled barbs she clung to. She couldn't see which way was up or down, but she knew the air was getting lighter; her ears throbbed and she could hardly breathe for her nerves.

The bright white of the sun caught Yaniqui's eye and she realized the dragon wasn't just soaring away from Akar Evion's commerce center—she was going straight up in the sky! She was going to do the only thing that would kill herself and Yaniqui along with her. The dragon thought it was better for both of them to die, rather than be owned as slaves. The prideful nature of the species was going to be Yaniqui's doom.

Black spots appeared at the sides of her vision. She lost her grip and should have fallen from the dragon, spiraling toward the ground, wind ripping at her like a bird with a broken wing. But she didn't. She started with a jolt when she realized she wasn't clinging to the thick spines anymore. She was an idiot to think she would have been able to hold on through the dragon's massive temper tantrum. She wasn't smart enough to figure out what was going on, but she was smart enough to know she was an idiot.

Yaniqui had arrived on Akar Evion some eighty hours prior.
"Don't look like that, Yaniqui," Mr. Savini said as an attendant strapped her into her seat on the minicraft.
A buckle twisted into her side as the attendant pulled the strap and crudely dug a finger under it to see that the property was secure.
"Transitions can be...hard, but it will be over soon. You'll be settled into your new home or facility and all the unknowns will wash away. The unknowns are the hardest part, I gather."
When Yaniqui was told she'd be offered for sale, when she learned Maemi was already gone, she quickly discovered what happened when she didn't cooperate. Her living quarters had been downgraded and the food she received was no longer expressly ordered to her room but delivered once a day. Yaniqui was used to that. If they thought hunger would break her, they'd never worked on an agricultural planet. But like on 4,278, the break came when they started overworking her. A parade of employees with various ailments was brought to her. If Yaniqui refused, she was electrocuted. Betha came once a day to tell Yaniqui it could all fade away if she would only cooperate. That hurt because Yaniqui had begun to trust Betha, trusted her to look out for her in a new world. When confronted, Betha said that's exactly what she was doing.
Strength was something Yaniqui always thought was inherent in herself. But she learned otherwise. A strong person would have defied Akar and lived a miserable life, but Yaniqui didn't see the point. She finally told Betha she'd cooperate and within hours she was reinstated in her plush room. She didn't have freedom—she never had—but she was comfortable once more. And if she was barreling through space toward owners that would use her how they saw fit, maybe comfort was the only gift she could give herself before then. So, she cooperated with everything, the photographs, the samples, the interviews,

everything. She spent weeks fighting hard to appear neutral. Trustworthy. Even grateful.

But when confronted with Savini's smug face, she couldn't bite her tongue any longer.

"It's better to *know* scientists will experiment on my body—tear it apart even?"

"If that's who wins the auction, then yes. In the end, you'd be sedated, peaceful—more than most of us can hope for in our moment of death. And you'd be saving lives." Mr. Savini crouched down by her, the attendant now checking the console. "The moment your planetary protection died, you had to have known how your life would end. You're too unique, too valuable. Your situation is acute in all ways, yet service will be no harder for you than any other being, and you have the added benefit of knowing you could save countless beings. This isn't as big of a deal as you're making it out to be. We're auctioning a dragon today too—it's going to be quite the event. We've never done *that* before."

"You've sold other Wea Saavians?"

His gray eyes clouded. "There are…records. Thank your god you're not being sold to some fighting ring or low-level brothel. No one's going to hunt you across the steppes of a wild planet. Before all this is over, you're going to save many people. Let that be a comfort to you."

"Do you give this pep talk to all the women you sell?"

"Don't be ridiculous. We sell men and women equally as well as nonconforming genders. No, I was merely curious." His eyes locked on Yaniqui's one final time as he left the minicraft.

Yaniqui lowered her eyes. One final time. Whatever Mr. Savini did with his, he wasn't accompanying her to the planet surface. She could act soon.

All she saw of Akar Evion was fields of buildings swallowed by fields of grass. It reminded her of the plant seas of 4,278, but these were naturally sprawling, not organized into tight rows. Her room on Akar Evion was much bigger than the one on the craft but much the same in contents. Yaniqui barely slept—she'd already had so much passive leisure time on the ship, plus she had to stay awake or miss her opportunity. The important thing was she act only once. The important thing was she give them all of herself, until the exact moment she could take it back.

It came when Betha scanned into her room the morning of the sale. She was carrying a very beautiful brocade gown in a deep violet. Yaniqui waited in the bathroom, staring in the mirror as she always did now when Betha came. Yaniqui stared into her own eyes. *You can do this.*

Her room was devoid of heavy objects except those bolted to the floor. There were blankets and towels because she was not a suicide risk. Since her change of heart weeks before, she tried to make it clear to Mr. Savini and everyone she interacted with that she valued her life too much to let a thing like slavery make her discard it.

It would come down to her fists. She was going to hit Betha in the face and steal her freedom.

Yaniqui exited the bathroom and realized beads of sweat had broken out along her spine. Her underarms weren't wet—they were drenched. She could smell her own fear. But when Betha turned and gave her a polite nod, Yaniqui smiled as if she didn't have a care in the world.

"This is the dress you'll wear for the auction." Betha raised her eyebrows. "It's going to be a good one—not just virtual. Some buyers have come in person."

"For me and the dragon too, I'm sure. It must be exciting, getting to see things like dragons."

"*Beings* like dragons," Betha corrected with a frown. "But large animoids are out in the warehouse district, not here. You're going to have to skip lunch today. When Emal comes, we'll go to the prep area. She'll bathe you and do your hair and makeup. Then we'll put this on."

"Oh," Yaniqui said, not disguising the fear in her voice.

Betha peered at her. "It will be fine. This is an easy process. You're pampered for the day and you'll wake up in a new exciting life tomorrow." She turned back to the task at hand. "And me," she said, "I get to clean your room. Thanks for not trashing it, by the way."

Betha typed in a code for a tiny cabinet in the wall and took a bottle of cleaner. She sprayed and wiped down surfaces starting on one side of the room. Then, she sprayed the surveillance camera. They were none too secret. Akar wanted you to know they were watching their property.

Yaniqui seized a tiny handheld vacuum and brought it down on Betha's turned head. The woman fell, the vacuum fell, and Yaniqui peered intently at the camera lens. She picked up the bottle of spray and sent another stream of foam for good measure. There was no time to check the woman's pulse, but she felt alive as Yaniqui stole her scan card, name badge, and stripped her of her white coat. Yaniqui had dressed in the plainest clothes she could find that morning, which were light-colored pants and a long-sleeve blouse. She was out the door in less than a minute, but already she knew it was too long. She hustled along a corridor, then another, and another. Door after door after door appeared. How many were filled with other trapped people like herself?

Finally, there was a transporter. Yaniqui calmly walked in behind two attendants dressed like Betha, and now herself. She rode down to the lowest level. There were no plush carpets and flickering light displays. The transporter doors opened to reveal cement floors. Dirty streaks showed on the walls. This was where Akar kept their own slaves.

Yaniqui followed the hall, then cut aside. She had little sense of the building but walked confidently and tried to tune in to her best instincts. She found the kitchen busy with men and women of all races chopping food. Fragrant steam hit her face but it only served to ignite her nerves and make her nauseous. One counter was clearly making upscale food for the guests—for her potential buyers. She found a loading dock for bringing fresh supplies in, looked around, and jumped down from the waist-high ledge.

It had to be known she was gone from her room by now. Someone would have checked the camera or maybe Betha was awake. Groggy, Yaniqui hoped. If Betha was alive, she would do her job.

Outside the loading dock, Yaniqui stashed the white jacket but slipped the nametag in her pocket. She grabbed a small crate at random as cover and walked down the wide alley, looking for any kind of garage with vehicles. Ideally, she'd hide herself in a craft and get off-planet before a thorough search was conducted for Akar's lost asset.

The weather was colder than she expected. The light-colored grasslands were deceptive. It was summer on-planet but frightfully cold waves blew through the gaps between buildings like a wind tunnel. The cloth under her wet arms went stark cold and Yaniqui knew she'd be shivering in minutes. Even chilled, even totally bewildered as to what she would do next, there was a certain pleasure in walking where no one knew where she was. Having a moment of pure autonomy was enough to keep her moving. She stole a look at the sky and saw a bird high above her.

Yaniqui ducked her head inside a hopeful-looking truck entrance and—yes!—it was a garage with a tiny, one-person hovercraft. She had no idea how to drive the vehicle. She hadn't driven anything since her Domi let her do a few trial runs as a kid. She sat on the hovercraft, currently flat on the floor, and patted it for keys or an ignition. The screen sprang to life. Of course, it required a key card or thumbprint with permissions.

"What are you doing?"

A lean man stood paces from Yaniqui. She was taken aback by his sudden appearance and then by the dark, swollen skin around one eye. Smoke trailed from his fingers and she realized he had snuck away to the garage to smoke undetected.

"I'm taking a ride."

Despite the situation, the man smiled. "I think you must be in the wrong place, miss, and definitely making the wrong decision. What you're about to do is going to get you killed. Are you from the kitchens?"

"Accounting, actually."

He raised his eyebrows and his umber forehead wrinkled except around the puffy eye. "I work in accounting. But I usually come down for lunch with a friend."

"Can you start this?" Yaniqui asked.

"It will do you no good. There's nowhere to go. And the short grass makes it impossible to hide."

Yaniqui threw everything to destiny. "I'm trying to escape. I can heal your eye. We can go together. Fate will protect us."

The man leaned down. Yaniqui reached for his face. He caught her hand in his. "Protect *you*, maybe," he whispered, "but sure, heal my eye, Wea Saavian."

Yaniqui's fingers warmed and felt the stickiness of pus. Her blood thrummed hesitantly from the light work.

The man touched his brow. "It's…sensitive."

"That will fade. Now come on."

He shook his head slowly. "I've got a better plan than yours. We need a diversion. Ever heard of a dŏsvengar?"

# Chapter 21
Lozen
The Catchment, Earth

At dawn, totally grumpy, chilled, and absolutely pissed off, Lozen squatted inside the tree line. The ground was damp with dew so she tried to keep her bottom clear of any wet leaves. She felt inside her bag for the device the agent had left her with. It was a handheld of some type. As soon as her eyes settled on the transponder, numbers and letters appeared. Despite herself, a thrill went through her.

She turned the transponder slowly in her hands. She wasn't stupid. She knew eye motion navigated it, but she had never seen one up close and the text was overwhelming. Further, though she could read signs and packaging and other basic things, she wasn't fully literate, especially when it came to new words. Lozen tested the device by moving herself around. The picture changed and she saw two red dots.

She stood and started out at a brisk pace. One of the markers shifted. Intent on watching the red dot move, she crashed over a fallen tree branch and fell. Her free hand squished in cold mud.

"Fucking capital idiots," Lozen swore. The agent wasn't the one that made her fall, but Lozen felt resentful toward her nonetheless. It was her fault Lozen was out there.

Lozen started again, walking this time, and followed the dot. It was not a long walk. If the GIA agent wanted to keep things quiet, she should have gone deeper into the woods. Everyone knew this inner perimeter was where teens snuck off to have sex. It was as likely that Lozen would trip over two bodies squashed together in a blanket as it was she would find the agent.

Soon it seemed the two dots would meet on the screen. She turned her attention to the trees in front of her and crept quietly until she could see who was waiting for her. It was definitely the man and woman from the blast site.

Most of the capital idiots were soft from such an easy life, but Lozen could see even at that distance the man was well muscled. Not quite good-looking, though she was sure he thought so. He read a holo tablet. Images and text shimmered around him. The woman carried an identical handheld to the one Lozen had. She looked at it, then straight at Lozen and waved her over. Lozen would have rather faced Lin and his matchmaking offers again, but she forced herself to leave the trees that sheltered her and marched forward, chin stuck out. The sooner she could get rid of the device, the sooner she'd have her privacy back.

All the same, Lozen approached them warily. She took care when she woke to braid her hair so there was no chance of her shorn stripe showing.

"We're from the GIA," the woman said, no greeting necessary. Her high ponytail pulled slightly at her temples and the small holo covering her shoulder scrolled an official-looking piece of literature, a disclaimer of some sort. "I'm Agent Tril."

"Agent Velazquez," the man said, looking up only briefly.

Both agents stood significantly taller than Lozen. Tril wasn't as athletic-looking as Velazquez, but she was much more severe.

"We're in the process of locating a perpetrator and we know you can help."

Lozen shook her head slightly, nervous to make any sudden movements around the agents. "I can't help you. I only came to return this device," she replied. She wished she didn't sound like a little girl.

No one made a move to take the transponder from Lozen's

outstretched hand. The woman continued as if Lozen hadn't spoken. "We set up mini cams at the bombing site. You stayed a long time, looking through the rubble for something. That wasn't the first time you'd been there. What are you looking for?"

"I was looking for supplies. Things that got left behind." Lozen was shaking, but suddenly everything clicked into focus. "Why are you interested in the bombing site? What do you know about what happened there?"

Tril ignored Lozen's questions and continued down her own train of thought. "We also know you met with Lin later that day."

Lozen cleared her throat.

"Of course, we keep tabs on Lin," Agent Tril said, answering the unspoken question. "It'd be nice if we knew what was said in all those meetings, but he's fastidious about sweeping his place."

"We can help you." Agent Velazquez stretched his neck while he took his turn talking. "You seem like a bright Earth girl. Let us take you out of the Catchment. Get you back to school so you can find a good job."

"Sure, I bet you have a pony too."

Like Tril, he continued as if Lozen hadn't spoken. "But first we need your help."

An image sprang from his holo: an ugly brown-orange beast with huge, powerful arms. It was hard to keep from recoiling. The holo spun slowly. It was clear the animoid was immense by any standard. Large, smooth shells ran down its arms and legs and a compilation of shell made its torso look like armor. Bristles peppered here and there but grew thickest on its elbows, knees, and shoulders that came up high, hiding the neck altogether. Soft ridges lined the bridge of the nose and they crinkled when the beast barred its broad teeth.

"We're looking for this D-68. He was picked up on Linkos after leading a large-scale operation against our miners there. Once apprehended, he killed a man, so he was taken to Earth for a trial. We have reason to think he bombed Station 9."

As he talked, Lozen's mind raced. In the past five minutes, she learned more about the bomber than she had in weeks. If she could bring this information to the Karmas, finish her initiation... She snapped to attention, memorizing everything she could about the disgusting creature.

Agent Tril said, "Lozen, this could be the most important thing you ever do. If you help us catch this guy, we'll make sure you never see the Catchment again. We'll set you up in the capital."

"What? You don't even know if that's what I want."

Velazquez cut his eyes in the direction of the Catchment and Lozen could read his mind. *Who wouldn't want to leave?*

Lozen rolled her eyes. "And this D-68, he, what, bombed the handout station from prison?"

Tril's mouth puckered before answering. "No. He escaped shortly after arriving on Earth."

Lozen was grateful for the information, but there was no way she was going to be caught working with the GIA by Lin or the Karmas.

"No thanks," she said. She made to give the transponder back—*just take it already*—when Velazquez typed something on his holo. A picture of a baby appeared, one with a lip more mangled than Lozen.

Lozen shot a dark look at the agents and then away at the trees. "I know how I look. And, gods, it's really not that big of a deal. I bet you'd kill to have hair like mine."

"Hang on here, look. Look."

It was the same baby, but the lip was perfect.

"We'll get that surgery for you. You just have to help us."

Lozen hated herself for it, but she felt her throat tighten with emotion. "But I don't know what to do or if I want to leave. I don't even know how to use this device. I-I-I can't read well," Lozen confessed.

"All you have to do," Tril said earnestly, "is be our eyes in the Catchment. It's difficult for us to move around here. All we're asking is that you report any signs of D-68 to us. It's a pretty easy exchange for a brand-new life."

Lozen pushed away a branch, frustrated, and it snapped back at her face. The sharp pain made her cry out, more of a gasp than a shriek, and she rubbed her skin until it was bearable. Her temper was high after creeping around the woods, looking for that animoid again, against her better judgment.

It had been days since she had met Tril and Velazquez, and Lozen still didn't know who she was really working for: the Karmas or the GIA. If she helped the Karmas, she'd be initiated in, part of a real community but stuck in poverty. If she helped the GIA, she'd leave the Catchment with a brand-new face, but she'd have to leave behind everything, including Monte. And if it was ever learned she was even in talks with the GIA, the government organization so many locals despised, she would be outed.

Both groups put their faith in Lozen and they shouldn't have bothered. Now she knew who the bomber was. As if that meant anything when she didn't have any other leads to go off.

But she didn't need to make any decisions until she knew *where* he was—if she could ever figure that out. It was better to wait and see how things developed. She wanted to support her new friends, but the offer of surgery was too compelling to give up easily.

Lozen passed a small hole in the ground and wished she were a chipmunk, hidden away from people and aliens. She was good at collecting acorns. If only that's all life took.

She drank heavily from her water bag. She wiped her mouth and, not for the first time, her heart sped as she imagined D-68 watching her through the budding dogwood branches. She used to be totally at ease in the forest, but ever since she saw the holo relay of D-68, the animoid haunted her thoughts. She imagined his huge frame moving silently through the brush, concealed until he came up right behind her.

Something rustled.

She whipped around and scanned the pattern of branches and dappled light. The budding leaves made it more difficult to see than in the winter. Dead leaves blew haphazardly along the moldering forest floor. She trembled a little, despite the spring weather.

Lozen changed direction. Apparently, she wasn't going to stumble upon D-68 in the woods, not that she wanted to.

Still, she didn't believe he had stayed in the Catchment—he was too large and different. Word would have gotten out. It occurred to her that even if he wasn't directly in the Catchment, the GIA was convinced he was here somewhere, which meant some*thing* had to know about him. Some animoid.

Her desire to complete initiation pushed her to return to the Catchment and then walk until the houses looked strange. Some structures were more rubble than house, others were groups of shacks in inward-facing circles. Orange stakes outlined a bare patch of tunneled ground. A group of flabby beasts wallowed in a drying mud patch with donated supplies scattered around them.

A large animoid with skin like a hairless cat walked on four limbs along the path, but two tiny—useless?—limbs hung from its sides. She looked away, as if someone's nakedness was exposed and the animoid did the same. Lozen bristled, offended at the thought that she looked as strange to it as it did to her.

Something caught Lozen's eye. Thinly shaved meat hung from a line, drying in the sun. The strips were large. The length of a child's arm? Monte's story flashed in her mind. Lozen forced her body not to turn and run. If she did that, she may as well be done. For the rest of her life. This was her one shot, one way or another.

Her heart leaped when she saw two humanoid men. Then they entered a building marked by a painted circle around a circle. They were there for sex.

Lozen wandered for some time, striving to look confident. Eventually, she came across a market made up of small shacks. Instead of a large ring or grid pattern like at the human markets, the tables and covered huts were bunched casually in the clearing. Some faced west, others grouped tightly together looking east. Lozen saw few food items and too many government handouts. It seemed no one wanted the purple coats.

At random, Lozen walked up to a female with thick teeth like a horse and a long neck though her shoulders and arms looked similar enough to an Earthling's. The animoid stood three heads taller than Lozen and bent her neck to talk to the human.

"I was told the price for coats was low," Lozen said, improvising.

The animoid said, "It is no secret we have many of these useless things. I cannot pretend to haggle. Take as many of these damn things as you like, but give me something more useful."

Lozen pretended to rummage through her bag, while looking

around the square. A few aliens watched back, but the rest went about their business as if she wasn't there.

"Will you take these?" Lozen asked, holding out several coins.

The animoid snatched them out of her hand—it acted like a person, but Lozen had trouble thinking of it that way—and prodded the coats in her direction. Lozen sorted through them, pretending to look at the size tags.

"Has the bombing affected the animoid blocks?" Lozen asked.

The animal shook her head. "It's too bad about yours. Tell your people to come here. To this market. We can make good deals," she cackled.

Lozen asked casually, "Are there other markets? Other places to get things?"

"Drug-e?"

Lozen shook her head quickly.

The female made a quick movement with her two hands that made a squelching noise.

"No. No. Um, are there those who know things?"

The animoid nodded at a human child sleeping under one of the tables. Lozen took a coat she didn't need and walked over, stomach going sour. What was one of her kind doing there? She bent down, but the child continued sleeping. She looked back at the thick-toothed woman, who mimed a tap.

Lozen touched the child's upper arm. Without preamble, he left the market and Lozen followed. She peeked once behind her and saw the vendor watching, face blank.

It felt safer with a guide, even one as frail and small as the boy. He brought her to a very small, neat house. The animoid equivalent of Lin. There was no line of others waiting for an audience, no one to pat her down. Lozen ducked to go in. It was dim and strangely clammy inside. Her eyes slowly adjusted. Three sacks stood in one corner. If it was food, it was an almost unheard-of amount. Dangerous too. It would be an immediate target for others.

Lozen turned her head.

She jumped back, her heart in her throat. Lozen shuddered as she took in the sight of a gigantic insect. It looked like a huge centipede, with a meaty but long body, and spindly legs shooting off from every part.

It *tsked tsked tsked.*

Lozen's skin crawled and she put her arms around herself. She would have run, but she felt as cold as lake ice.

The boy translated, "He said don't be so rude." The boy spoke smoothly, even confidently. "He's rather good-looking where he's from. You don't look that great, besides." His words broke the film over the surface. Lozen felt not better but sane.

"And you are?"

The boy responded, no translation necessary, "You can call him Leggs."

If Lozen wasn't so terrified and grossed out, she would have rolled her eyes. Unless he was poisonous or deadly in another way, Lozen could not see why anyone would look to him as a boss. Why would he warrant respect in a village of larger-than-life characters? Who would give him information and come to him for help?

"I'm looking for someone."

Leggs *tsked* and the boy spoke. "Aren't we all, child?"

If Lozen could have understood Leggs's tone, she would have wondered if it was wistful or sarcastic.

"An alien animoid. He might go by the name D-68. Very large, rust in color, with huge shoulders and arms."

Leggs's many legs trembled as he walked slowly up the side of the wall and peered out a large crack near the ceiling. He turned his oblong head her way. "I've never heard the name D-68, but I've heard rumors of someone by that description. Whether or not he's in the Catchment, well…"

"I can offer you a lot. I could—I could assure that you'd receive better accommodations. More food."

*Tsk tsk.*

"It's true, this house is too drafty for my kind. In the winters, I suffer greatly. But are you not just a human girl from the Catchment?"

"I have a powerful benefactor," Lozen said. She knew she didn't look like someone who would have any influence.

"The GIA?" the boy asked.

Lozen shrugged.

"And what about this other-worlder? If I reveal his location, will I be responsible for his death?"

"D-68 escaped from his impending trial. All I know is there have been charges brought against him. And you know about the bombing in the humanoid block."

The boy's face was blank as he translated. "Terrible atrocities. I would like to bring this monster to justice for killing Earthlings after they've shared their world with us. However, I will need more than food and blankets I do not use. I want a trip to the outside. I want to see the capital."

# Chapter 22

Adam
In Transit

When the monster was well out of sight, Eeriva let Hloban off the floor with threats of what would happen if he did anything to call the beast's attention to them again. Adam could only assume Hloban had had a complete psychotic break—how else could someone fathom willingly calling out to that dragon? Adam himself was still shaking with fear and useless adrenaline. He tried to rub life back into his numb limbs. Keyad and Waquas spoke in low tones about the wisdom of waiting for the skies to clear before leaving the atmosphere. No one asked Adam, but he agreed.

"Mission failure." Eeriva rubbed both hands slowly over her eyes. "I'll let Cortez's office know we're heading back to Earth."

Hloban stood half-bent at a porthole, straining to stare up at the clear sky. Thin clouds of ship exhaust and dust streaked the blue, but there was no sign of Yaniqui. At the mention of Earth, Hloban snapped out of his reprieve.

"What are you talking about? Of course, we're going to follow Yaniqui." He looked each of his companions in the face, incredulous.

"That's why we came all this way!"

"Hloban, you can't be serious. Coming here was a bad call. The dragon made the situation a hundred times more dangerous than we ever expected and, she's—" Everyone looked at Eeriva as she faltered. "I mean, she couldn't—well, Hloban, she's no longer with us."

Hloban looked up at the ceiling in frustration, as he if could hardly stand the sight of Eeriva's tiny head and tiny thoughts. "The dragon could have set her down. She was *obviously* working with that beast as a team."

"Then she didn't need us to save her," Eeriva said.

Hloban opened his mouth.

"No, Hloban, I don't want to hear it. I'm sorry she's gone, but there is nothing anyone can do now."

Waquas spoke, "Hloban, this is a good thing. She was resourceful enough to find her way out of captivity and climb on the back of a dragon." He paused until Hloban looked at him. "Eeriva's right. *If* she's alive, she certainly doesn't need our help. She's hopefully going to get as far away as she possibly can, go into hiding, and live a long, safe life."

Hloban couldn't hold it back any longer. "But Yaniqui will never even know we were here. She will never know how close I was. If I had gotten to her sooner, she'd be on the *Caneille* now." He started crying. "I'll never see her again."

Eeriva pulled out the stack of holo maps to draft the journey back to Earth and plugged one into the console. Waquas guided the *Caneille* up toward the atmosphere—in the opposite direction as the dragon. Eeriva asked Waquas a question every once in a while to clarify their path.

Only Adam's dad seemed sympathetic to Hloban's misery and sat with his arm around his friend. The thought shocked Adam. He didn't think of Hloban and his dad as friends—rather that they were the last of their kind stuck on the same planet. His dad had always been a little shy, and definitely on the outskirts of the real scene in the capital. Hloban was the opposite. He was bold and made himself welcome in anything he wanted to. He was arrogant, but Adam admired him. He was similar to Loera in that way: overconfident but incredibly likeable.

Which was why, later, Adam told his dad privately in the dorm it was probably better this way.

"I never understood the plan to relocate Yaniqui to Earth and then just, what? Hope Yaniqui and Loera went to spin class together?"

"People are complex, Adam. Sometimes we can only act and wait for fate to take over."

Adam's retort was immediate. "Don't give me that. That's nothing more than 'hoping for the best' and that hardly works out on its own."

His dad reminded him that he grew up on Earth. He didn't understand Hloban's link to Yaniqui. Plus, Adam had never loved someone before. When he noticed Adam's sour expression, his dad laughed and asked if he wanted to fight a dragon for a girl too.

"No, of course not." Adam hesitated. "It's just…now we have to go home."

"You're upset about failing? Consider how much closure we brought Hloban—he got to see his betrothed one last time."

"Before she crisped up in the atmosphere?" He saw his dad was distantly uncomfortable and apologized. "It's not that. I know it's selfish, but what about me? I'm returning to Earth with nothing."

"You've now been to space, on your first boost even."

"Yeah," he mumbled.

Keyad searched the Wave for news of the dragon, but he could not find any mention or sign of it or Yaniqui's whereabouts. There wasn't even a notice that the auction was canceled. Akar simply didn't mention anything about their warehouse blowing up, the dozens of ships taken out by a rare, evidently unwilling, captive dragon, or the escape of what Akar had called "the being that can heal the medical system." The larger galaxy would think the auction had taken place, and no law-abiding civilians but them would ever know the truth. Hloban sat dejectedly at the table and showed no interest in any of it.

Waquas suggested spending ship energy on a call home to Loera, but Hloban ate a fishy-smelling meal bar instead and lay over the side of the table. It was so uncomely, it inspired Adam to shake off his own gloomy attitude.

Adam was being too hard on himself. He wondered how many

people in the galaxy could say they saw a dragon in the midst of a battle and survived. Ideas flitted through his head. The intro to an interstellar travel book. Interviews on Earth. Interviews on the Jupiter Station. Briefings on the security threat dragons posed to Earth. It could give him the funding to get off Earth again. Then, the spark took hold…it was too vast. There were too many things to think about. Could he find more dragons and become an expert? For the first time, he considered that Yaniqui might still be alive—it was better for his narrative if she was. And if she had convinced the dragon to save her, what could he do?

With all of these ideas, it felt almost like he had already done it all. He just had to go through the motions to make it real.

Keyad finished with the wall screen so Adam sat in front of it and looked up information on dragons. They were animoids, one of the Original Nine species and the only one not to break off into subspecies. It was thought that they were the oldest species with a consciousness in the galaxy. Their fire was made up of caesium and hydrogen, which was why it was so notoriously hard to put out.

They had evolved the ability to leave their origin planet and travel through space. Tiny tardigrades and huge dragons were the only animoids that could survive in a vacuum. Dragons are impervious to extreme temperatures and can go great lengths without breathing. Adam wondered about that. Yaniqui had a jumpsuit and helmet but neither of those would be anywhere near enough to withstand the speed required to escape Akar Evion's gravity and soar through space. The temperature, the radiation…there were a hundred ways to die.

Something tiny burst inside Adam when he realized Yaniqui was dead after all.

Dragon physiology was fascinating, but the rest of the reading was sad. Dragons had ruled the galaxy for eons, spreading slowly from one planet to the next over millennia, unlike humanoids who conquered star systems in the span of lifetimes. The Black Wars was a dark period when it seemed like dragons would stamp out the invasive vermin they saw humanoids to be for overreaching, constantly conquering, and wiping out entire ecosystems. But, like ants, humans repopulated quicker than dragons.

Few dragons were left and those were notoriously difficult to contact. They had no delegate in the Joint Council and did not allow any other species to involve themselves in dragon affairs.

Suddenly, the screen went black. "This isn't just to look stuff up on," his dad said and shooed him off. "The data downloads cost money."

Adam ran on the treadmill and drank a packet of water before dusting himself down to get the sweat off. He was eager for a real shower.

He replayed Yaniqui's escape and all the information he had learned. One thing bothered him. How did the dragon get away from Akar Evion without detection if it couldn't go light speed like a ship? And how did dragons travel far enough to populate other worlds, if not with technology?

The articles made it clear in addition to rapidly repopulating, the other thing that turned the Black Wars was human technology. Unlike nearly every other form of Intelligent life that had innate instinct and abilities, humans were obsessed with creating machinery and equipment to achieve their goals and expand their territory.

It was thought that dragons went into a type of stasis as they drifted through space until they neared another planet. But that had to be dangerous, even for a being such as a dragon. And no one ever just stumbled upon a dragon floating through space, did they?

Adam slipped his underwear on and ran out of the bathroom, still dusty.

"Asteroids," he said.

Waquas did a double take at the monitor on the console and then smiled warily at Adam.

"Finish dusting off and go to bed," his dad said kindly.

"No, no. I've got it. Dragons move around the galaxy, but they don't use technology and they can't fly on their own for such large distances. Dragons must asteroid-hop. It would conserve energy, protect them from radiation, and camouflage themselves from human technology. I bet that dragon is on an asteroid and, well, *maybe* Yaniqui too."

His dad and Waquas looked at each other. At the sound of

Yaniqui's name, Hloban jolted to the holo and pulled up a shared info collection of known asteroids and comets, accessible for travelers.

Keyad woke Eeriva who rolled her eyes but Adam kept pushing. Hloban would believe anything that could bring them to Yaniqui so the real approval came from Waquas.

"Look," he said, pointing at the display, "there was an asteroid within relative distance of Evion."

"And so, what if there was?" Eeriva demanded. "Waquas, we can't go anywhere near a dragon. And Yaniqui's not going to be alive!"

"I think the dragon saved her," Adam said. "I think she knew the dragon was her best shot at getting off-planet and they saved each other. I don't think it would just eat her afterward."

"You read one article and now you're an expert?"

Adam heard the disdain in Eeriva's voice, but shrugged and said, "They're incredibly powerful beings, but they have to have a way to transport their young through space."

"They lay eggs."

"Well, I don't know everything! But it's worth a shot!"

They took a vote. Eeriva was the only one that voted against pursuing the asteroid because, as she said, the girl was dead.

Things were tense as they shifted course. It was eventually decided they would not use the cloaking device. The dragon would know they were there, and Adam said honesty was important when dealing with dragons. Eeriva snorted again.

Waquas brought them in toward the asteroid cautiously, as the ship was jumpy so near an unstable source of gravity. Adam peered at the side camera monitors. The asteroid looked like those in the belt between Mars and Jupiter, all gray and pockmarked. It was a barren hunk of minerals and metals with no atmosphere. Waquas ran calculations and the data showed this one was one and a half miles long. He did a heat scan, but there was nothing. Eeriva groaned, but Waquas set a route to take them across and around the asteroid in a grid pattern. Visual confirmation would be painstaking work, but it was the only way.

Adam was committed to seeing the whole thing through as it was his idea, but the others took shifts watching the cameras.

Then...

"Fuck yes," Hloban said.

Everyone crowded around as Waquas brought the ship in parallel to a ridge.

"How is she able to withstand the force and temperatures? She should be dead," Eeriva exclaimed.

"She's close to the dragon," Adam said with a smile. "There's some reason they can survive in space. She's leeching off that somehow."

"They're working together," his dad corrected.

The *Caneille* jarred slightly as Waquas landed on the unstable surface with the larger of the two portholes facing the dragon. Hloban stood squarely in the viewpoint, but upon impact, a blanket of dust rose slowly around them, obscuring their sight. When it cleared, the dragon was up on all four legs, its neck arching back and forth as it took the ship in. The beast smoldered and Adam remembered the images of ships twisting and melting in on themselves.

He caught sight of Hloban's face and the emotion there was too much for Adam to bear looking at. The hope was too vulnerable to see in a proper adult.

On the screen, Adam saw the helmeted Yaniqui watching the ship. The dragon put its large head down by Yaniqui, keeping both eyes on the craft.

*Come on*, Adam thought impatiently. What was she waiting for?

With sudden inspiration, Adam pulled his dad over to the window and made sure all three of them were visible. One is easier to fake than three.

Yaniqui turned and said something to the dragon, visor still masking her features. They seemed to confer.

"Ehhh, this is bad. This was a bad idea," Eeriva said.

The crew paused, every motion or breath sure to set off the immense creature.

Yaniqui kept a hand on the dragon as they approached the spaceship. She disappeared from view as the pair closed the distance. Soon it was just the dragon, eyes locked on Adam and the other Wea

Saavians. With no facial cues, there was no way to tell what the dragon thought or felt. The skin wasn't flat black. In the glow of the ship's lights, it looked purple at times, then dark blue.

*Memorize all of this,* Adam told himself.

The dragon's snout pressed against the window and Adam stepped back. There was no condensation or breath. It lowered its giant head and peered in with one molten eye. Everyone froze. The eye saw all. Adam's skin crawled and sweat broke out on his neck. For one wild moment, he wondered if he was actually going to piss his pants. Waquas put a hand up, reaching toward the dragon, seemingly without knowing he did so.

Finally, the dragon's head disappeared. A sharp rasp sounded against the belly of the *Caneille.*

"Fuck," Eeriva whispered.

Hloban jerked to attention, as if out of a daze, and went to the control panel. The ship hummed as it lowered the ramp to the air lock doors. On-camera, they could see Yaniqui ascend the ramp and step through the first set of doors.

The dragon glided a short distance—not with its wings out, but as a leap supported by the soft gravity—and curled its neck to rest, eyes still trained forward.

Hloban sprinted to the back room and everyone followed in a rush.

# Chapter 23
## Yaniqui In Transit

The doors behind Yaniqui slid shut and she felt the pull of artificial gravity and air pressure readjust. Her breath came fast with nerves and she swallowed. The doors in front of her slid open and she stepped into a hall crowded with the craft's crew. She cast her eyes frantically across the lot for some clue as to who these people were and how they had found her. A man with skin the color of a new leaf stepped aside to allow the rest see around his tall frame.

"Yaniqui?" someone asked quietly.

Oh gods. Black hair, golden skin. It was true. They were Wea Saavian. And they had come for *her*. She was found. She blinked quickly to stem the tide of tears and sniffed as she undid the clasps on the helmet and pulled it off. Her ears popped. She could only imagine how she looked with scorch marks and crystalized frost in equal measure across her suit. Her hair hung thick with dried sweat. She had no sense of how much time had passed since she was on Akar Evion waiting to be sold, but she had been through quite a bit since she last bathed.

"Who are you?"

"You're safe," a man blurted and broke out in a huge grin. "You're finally safe." His black hair lay in rumpled layers, not quite long enough to be curls. His brows were dark as well and lay thick but well-groomed over deep brown eyes. The man straightened, steeling himself in the face of what he was about to say. "Yani, it's me—Hloban."

Stars crashed.

An electric current ran through Yaniqui's body and her mouth dropped. She blinked and studied his face for a hint of the boy she knew a decade ago. He nodded in response, intent on her, drinking in her own face like a languid pool of water in a dry desert. She laughed and suddenly her body launched forward in sheer delight. She threw herself on Hloban, hugging him and laughing.

He felt perfectly made for her as their bodies connected. Yaniqui felt the twisting thrill of desire bloom. She leaned forward and kissed him. A dark heat stole over her mouth and she pushed herself against him harder. Life welled up inside her. It was incredible and confounding. A slight break in the kiss brought a humid breath. Then they were kissing again and she felt her entire body awaken to the life she had spent a decade longing for.

Someone sniffed loudly and Hloban pushed lightly on her shoulders and they broke apart. She found the others openly gawking at them. Yaniqui blushed but realized she didn't care. It was the best day of her life.

Hloban beamed. "I can't believe it, Yaniqui." He turned to the rest of the crew. "We did it, you guys!" He bounced with energy. "I'd like you to meet Yaniqui. This is Keyad," Hloban said, pointing out a middle-aged man. "He's Wea Saavian too. That's his son, Adam, who grew up on Earth."

"Hey." Adam waved in shock and cleared his throat nervously. It was clear he was part Wea Saavian, but something else as well.

Both of the men were taller than Hloban who was nearly exactly Yaniqui's height. As if he couldn't get any more perfect.

"You're full Wea Saavian?" Yaniqui asked, looking at the man. "How did you escape the solar flare?"

"I was already living on Earth at the time."

Yaniqui tilted her head. "Living on another planet?"

Keyad nodded, expecting her surprise. "I left Wea Saa many years before the flare, but I missed, and still miss, it every day. I'll tell you about it sometime."

Yaniqui was about to ask a follow-up question despite Keyad's promise to tell the story another time when Hloban introduced the tallest man as Waquas and a strong, determined-looking woman as Eeriva. While Eeriva was dressed in a standard jumpsuit, the rest were in casual clothes.

"Eeriva?" Yaniqui asked carefully. "I knew a cook named Zimetta. Those are both Klevan names, right?"

The woman shook a shaggy head of hair. Most of her hair was emerald but the wide part was fair. "No, I'm from Earth. That's where we all came from." Her strong, bouncy accent stood out among the others' speech and though Yaniqui's smile was the widest it'd ever been, it stretched a little more.

Waquas reached out and took Yaniqui's hand in his. "We didn't think we'd find you again after Evion."

His hand was warm. Yaniqui just noticed how cold she really was and shivered.

It would have been impolite to ask, but Yaniqui wondered what Waquas's role was in the group. With green skin and hairless brows, he obviously wasn't Wea Saavian or an Earthling. Though the back hall was tangled with tensions of all kinds, he radiated calmness.

"I didn't expect to be found."

Hloban's face clouded and she felt his grip on her arm tighten. Good. Yaniqui had so many questions about Earth and who everyone was and how they came to be in the exact right place at the exact right time. Was this how fate worked? Was she finally experiencing the promise of her people?

Yaniqui looked around the room. "Thank you for saving me and reuniting me with Hloban."

The last sentence seemed to signal to everyone that they should go back to their normal routines so they drifted down the hall and came out in the main living area. The cockpit sat at the front. The craft was as small as Yaniqui guessed from the outside. Full-spectrum lightbulbs lit rows of lush green plants growing in bubbling water. The seats at the console looked worn and cracked and one of the overhead lights buzzed, but after the plush accommodations of Akar, there couldn't have been anything better.

Eeriva offered Yaniqui a shower, but she couldn't bear to leave Hloban's side. Not at first. She did accept some food from Keyad and sat opposite the table from Hloban. The others seemed to converge in one corner of the mains, giving them some semblance of privacy. It was fairly ordinary. The only thing that stuck out was an ugly unholstered couch bolted to the floor. Adam whispered something to his dad.

She took her first bite as if her life depended on it and smiled, mouth closed while she chewed. She realized how incredibly sapped of energy her body was and took another hungry bite. Hloban looked like so much more than she remembered. His dark hair was only long enough to stand in a bristly patch, curls not long enough to form. Black lashes lined his eyes. He had angular cheekbones and impossibly smooth skin.

And his voice. Yaniqui had waited her whole life to hear his voice again.

"We were on Akar Evion."

She stopped chewing. "You were?"

Hloban nodded seriously. "We came to rescue you, but what you did was incredible."

Abruptly, Adam flopped down on the bench next to Hloban. He folded his arms across the table and peered at Yaniqui as if preparing for an interview. Yaniqui looked at Hloban in alarm.

"How did you live through it all? I mean, you should have died ten times in the past day," he said.

"The dŏsvengar has an inherent protective shield."

"Dŏsvengar?" Adam asked.

"It's what they call themselves. It spoke to me, but in my head, you know? I've never experienced anything like that." Yaniqui licked crumbs off a finger. "A force field protects them from the heat of their own blasts and the friction from entering and leaving atmospheres."

Hloban spoke, "But how would you have survived? Why did you go up with it into space? If you didn't die then, you would have eventually become oxygen-starved."

"I had planned to release the dŏsvengar as a distraction. Someone gave me the access code. It later occurred to me that I was *their* distraction. I was going to steal a craft, but she told me if I went with her I'd be saved. She's very persuasive." Yaniqui sighed. "I was starting to think she meant it in a redemption-through-death sense though. There's not much air left in this suit. It was like I was sleepy the entire time I was with her. She had been…closing in on herself. I guess you could say hibernating. When I made sense of what I was seeing on the asteroid, all of you, it was like I took a huge gulp of air and everything rushed to my head."

Adam had more questions—Yaniqui got the sense that he was about to start writing things down—when Hloban interrupted him. "Yaniqui needs to rest." He turned to his betrothed. "We can talk everything through tomorrow. You're safe now."

"Oh, that's right," Eeriva said from across the room. She opened one of the small lockers. "Here. We've had this bag for you since we left Earth. Loera packed a few supplies she thought you'd need." She handed the tiny bag to Yaniqui.

In her peripheral vision, Yaniqui saw Adam make eye contact with Waquas, who raised his nonexistent eyebrows. What was that about?

Yaniqui pulled out a clear, zippered plastic bag that held tiny cosmetic bottles.

Yaniqui pulled out a handful of clothes. They unraveled and slithered against each other. A pink shirt fell to the ground. Right away, she knew there was something wrong with the clothes, but she seized one anyway. Dropping the rest on the floor, no longer remotely tidy, Yaniqui stretched and held up a gray knit sweater. It was tiny and obviously juvenile, like something a fourteen-year-old might wear to school.

Keyad laughed. "Well, good thing we wasted supply space on that. Why would Loera have packed that?"

"Who's Loera?" Yaniqui asked.

"Balls," Hloban muttered. "It's fine," he said more clearly. "We'll get you something to wear."

But Eeriva was talking too. "This explains a lot." She barked a laugh that unsettled Yaniqui. "Loera's willingness to add another person to her household, her mild-tempered acceptance of the situation." She saw Yaniqui's confusion. "Hloban hasn't told you about Loera yet? You're going to *love* her."

Hloban shook his head at Eeriva, already standing from the bench. "Yani, I'll show you where you can lie down. You're exhausted."

"Everyone loves Loera," Eeriva said, exaggeratedly, "but Hloban loves her best, of course."

Yaniqui glanced up sharply at Hloban's face. "Who is she talking about?" She struggled to keep her voice even.

Hloban looked around the mains as if someone was going to help him. Adam licked his lips, ran his hand through his hair, and stood up too. Instinctively, Yaniqui knew this was going to be bad.

"Loera is, well, she's my wife."

Yaniqui's lips parted, less sensuously than before. She rose from her seat slowly. "You got married?"

"They have an adorable little boy too," Eeriva added.

Hloban shot a dark glare at Eeriva, but Yaniqui pushed him back by the shoulder, forcing him to look at her.

"You got married? Hloban, I don't understand." The universe was a dumpster fire. She couldn't breathe. "We were betrothed!" Oh crisps, she couldn't breathe!

Hloban turned slightly, as if he could block their audience, and lowered his voice. "We don't need to talk about this now—"

She opened her mouth but no words came out. She tried again. "I need to know—I need to know exactly what's going on."

Keyad had long since disappeared into another room and Waquas was intently chipping away at a dried brown stain on the control panel. Adam sat in the chair next to Waquas, moving carefully as if he could avoid calling notice to himself. Only Eeriva seemed undisturbed.

"Yaniqui, you need to breathe." He took an exaggerated breath and let it out in a quick *whoosh*. "Yes, I'm married. Her name is Loera. She's an Earthling. We have a son together. His name is Obani."

Hloban put both hands out, palms up, a peace offering. "We were betrothed, but we were young. And then I thought you were dead. I had no idea—no idea—you were still out there until Akar announced they had you. I couldn't leave you in their possession, and besides, the uh, leader of Earth really wants you to come there. But the most important thing is you're safe—"

He continued speaking, but Yaniqui was working something out in her head and she interrupted him. "Your kid's name is Obani?" she asked, fist clenched tight, shoulders taut under her spacesuit. "What an interesting name for you and *your wife* to choose. It's almost too traditional."

From across the way, Adam looked up with a gasp. Yaniqui couldn't help but round on him and glare, but she didn't have the time to cuss him out. She had to turn back to the matter at hand.

"And does *she* by chance think I'm some little teenager?" Yaniqui's head tilted as she looked at him in desperation.

"Probably," Eeriva said.

Hloban turned and made an X with his arms and opened them quickly as if he could expel Eeriva. "Please. Stop." He turned to Yaniqui and took another breath. He said with exaggerated calmness, "I told Loera a lot about you. She knows that we were destined—but that we were separated a long time ago. She does know that you were younger than me. Loera also knows you're someone who needs help, and she wants to help you. I don't know about the clothes."

Yaniqui let out a snort at this, part disbelief and part frustration.

Seizing the opening to finalize the matter once and for all, Hloban barreled on, "And I want to help you too."

Yaniqui's head cocked, her eyes squinted to a glare. "I can believe someone I've never met before might want to help me. But you?"

Hloban looked crestfallen and then angry.

"You haven't done a crisping thing since I was taken," Yaniqui said. "You didn't look for me. You didn't remember me." Her voice grew louder with each statement.

Waquas finally looked up, unable to continue pretending drama wasn't unfolding.

"You didn't care for me. You found another partner and went on with your life. I can't believe I thought our reunion was destiny.

"Just for a moment, I thought that after all of those terrible—" her voice broke "—hard things, we were finally going to be together. That the stars knew what they were doing after all. That linking us—two people who miraculously escaped the destruction of their planet—meant we would find each other again. Because we were supposed to be together."

"Can you guys stop it with the hand-holdy words?" Adam said.

The crisp was with that kid and that woman and everybody else? She seized the metal tray of meal bars and lunged at Adam's head.

# Chapter 24
## Hloban
## In Transit

Yaniqui took an extremely long shower—much to Eeriva's ire—and promptly hid herself away in the dormitory. Hloban was going on thirty hours without sleep, but you couldn't have paid him to go in there unaccompanied. Adam was still licking his wounds. Things couldn't have gone worse. Unless the Wipeout Con Hloban hidden after the disaster at Evion suddenly burst open and sucked the oxygen out of the room.

There was always that.

"What exactly is the plan when we get back to Earth with her?" Adam asked.

Hloban didn't respond. He sat on the couch, legs extended in front of him, eyes closed. Maybe if he pretended Adam didn't exist, he could fall asleep and everything would be better when he woke up.

"Maybe we should be glad we found her and she's safe now," Waquas said.

"Yeah, yeah, totally. But I mean, is she, like, going to live with Hloban and Loera?" As Hloban wasn't answering him, Adam was speaking as if Hloban wasn't there, though no one believed him to be asleep. "Is Hloban going to leave Loera for her? I didn't expect their reunion to be so…wet."

Eeriva sank into a chair next to Waquas but addressed the whole room. "Well, I for one am not going to stand by. Now that Yaniqui's safe, we can't let Hloban lose perspective. He already has a family."

"I don't know if it's our business," Waquas said.

"When you're on a ship together, everything is everyone's business."

It was working. The insufferable conversation felt more muted than the previous moment. *Please,* Hloban thought, *give me oblivion.*

For once, it was peaceful. There was no beep from the console warning the portside defrosters were sputtering with despair and condensation and preparing to freeze over, the first stop to death in space. Keyad and Eeriva weren't bickering over the dinner menu. Adam wasn't shooting human remains into space. And Yaniqui wasn't crying, throwing things, or screeching in the air lock.

Hloban batted his eyes open. He had fallen off the couch and his nose was currently squashed against the cold floor. He moved slowly to accommodate the crick in his neck.

He looked around and decided Yaniqui must still have domain over the dorm. Adam's voice came from the back hall as he muttered to himself and the hum of running water came from the bath capsule. Waquas was the only one missing so it must have been him showering.

Hloban rolled slowly up, picked up his hand device, and, after a moment's consideration of watching the Zarbon dramas everyone else on board hated, he clicked over to the library and selected Loera's reading list, as if that was what he intended to do all along.

*The 12 Steps of Essential Project Performance*

*A Leader Among Men*

*The Busy Life: Slice Your Schedule As Thin as Finely Shaved Prosciutto*

Loera's assistant stocked her reading list with the most current business books, but Hloban scrolled until he found a group of titles he knew Loera had downloaded herself. He clicked on *It's Over or It's*

*Eden.*

The first line was good, but that was as far as Hloban got.

Eeriva sat down closer on the couch than was strictly necessary. Especially if she just intended to relax—something she'd never heard of. No, she was sitting and sitting close. She had something to say.

Hloban wanted to know what the second paragraph said, so it seemed like a great time to be passive-aggressive. He wasn't going to look up until he could no longer reasonably ignore Eeriva.

Eeriva cleared her throat and Hloban pretended to scratch his jaw as he tried to read fast enough to get the basic premise of the book.

"Hloban," she finally said. "We need to talk. Everyone is miserable."

Hloban shot her a look out of the corner of his eye. "It seems peaceful to me."

"That's because your girlfriend is showering—again—and for once can't snap at all of us over your shortcomings as a lover."

His fingers tightened on the device. "Please don't exaggerate, Eeriva. She's not my girlfriend."

"Yeah, but she was."

"No," he stressed. He finally turned toward the executive officer. "She wasn't." He saw the look of disbelief on her face and countered it. "Look at our age difference. We were betrothed when she was born. I knew her and her family, but she was just starting her apprenticeship and I was near finishing mine. Our families vacationed together when we were little and we spent holidays together, but she had her friends and I had mine."

"And you didn't expect her to be all lovey-dovey?"

Hloban dodged the subject. What he expected was fraught with thoughts, ideas, and longings that were incompatible with each other. He still felt wildly guilty about the kiss, but that had just happened. He couldn't be responsible.

"Things are already cooling down, Eeriva. All is right in the galaxy. We saved a woman from human trafficking, Akar has no idea it was us, and now we're speeding toward whatever life you have on Earth. You gonna go on a hot date when we get back?"

Eeriva rolled her eyes. "That's personal."

Hloban had picked up the reader, looking for his place on the second page but put it back down incredulously. "Oh, that's personal, but what's between Yaniqui and me isn't?"

"No, it isn't. What's going on between you two affects the whole ship. And, if something bad should happen, we are not functioning as tightly as we should be. Your personal issues could jeopardize everyone's safety."

Hloban heard the bath capsule door slide open down the hall. Then, a very wet and very flushed Yaniqui stepped out wrapped in a towel. Her black curls hung limply at her shoulders, waiting for the opportunity to dry and spring up again.

"That water pressure is remarkable."

Eeriva looked slyly over at Hloban. "Only the best on Hloban's ship." She stood. "I better go do inventory."

Adam appeared in the doorway, arms full of bags of grain he brought from the back.

"Ohmigods, Yaniqui, put some clothes on."

Yaniqui, who had been gently beaming at Hloban for having such a nice spacecraft, turned her eyes on Adam. "Crisping heck, Adam. It's not a big deal. On 4,278, there was basically no divider where the men and women washed…outside. Naked!"

Keyad's shoulders stiffened. Hloban could sense he was telling himself not to turn around and busied himself with checking a reader on the console.

Where Yaniqui had been demure and pleasant moments ago, she now stood aggressively contrapposto, arms folded tightly across her chest.

"Oh sure, the labor planet," Adam said. "You're so much more worldly than me."

"Technically, I am," she said coldly. "I've been on more planets than you."

"By, like, one!"

Yaniqui pulled up her towel and Hloban wouldn't have been surprised if she bared her teeth.

"Hey, let's dial it back."

Yaniqui turned on Hloban. "What does that even mean, Hloban?"

Oh gods. She was so angry with him—clearly she was both happy to finally be together and furious at all he'd done while they were separated and one emotion hadn't won out over the other, but it didn't matter—no one could say his name like her. Literally. Keyad's Wea Saavian accent had weakened over time. Adam had none. Yaniqui could clearly hide hers but could also lay it on thick. So very thick. *Hthobennn.*

Heat rushed to his face and he looked aside. "It's an Earth phrase. Now, why don't you go get dressed?"

It was too late. And too the wrong thing to say to a woman in love with him.

"Oh, I'm sorry, Hloban. I didn't realize everyone on this craft was such a prude. Including the man who was supposed to be my husband!"

Yaniqui stormed to the dormitory and threw open the door. Out carried Waquas's bemused voice. Yaniqui spun on one heel and walked in the other direction. The only place she could go was back to the bath capsule.

Adam laughed. "No one else allowed to be half-naked around here?"

"Shut up," she hissed.

Waquas came out in only his briefs but was pulling a shirt on.

Eeriva returned, too keen to be left out of anything that happened, good or bad.

They all looked at Hloban.

"Yaniqui," he said hesitantly. "I'm just saying, there's not a lot of space, so let's respect each other's boundaries. And knock."

All was quiet. Even Yaniqui. She looked at him as if she'd never really seen him before. Her body tensed under the buildup of steam. Her wet hair was still plastered to her shoulders, but her humid, lustful look was gone.

"Boundaries!"

Ah, it seemed that snapping was going to be a regular thing from now on.

"You're the one who forgot about *boundaries*, Hloban! Marrying an Earthling? Forgetting about me and getting on with your life while

I worked and lived in squalid conditions and was nearly purchased by a company that wanted to scrape my guts out. And now we're flying on a craft to *your* new home planet where I'm going to waste away like some weird aunt to your kid, and you want to talk about boundaries?"

She didn't wait. She swept past Waquas who took a hasty half step back for fear of bumping against the humid mass of hate.

Hloban had so desperately wanted to be a hero to both women. Now, he was certain he was the villain.

The rest of Hloban's day cycle was tense and he couldn't help but think about what the journey back would have been like if he had just been able to keep news of Loera under wraps for another day. Two days tops. Maybe a week.

He could have heard Yaniqui's story in full and told her his plan to take care of her. Established some distance, cemented a quasi-sibling relationship before he told her he had definitively moved on. He may not have been married to Yaniqui, but his entire youth had been spent with that intention. The only reason he was with Loera was because he thought Yaniqui was dead. It was only keeping her memory alive that kept him searching for her.

Instead, Yaniqui and Adam bickered over whether she was being careful enough with his Earthling copy of a space travel book. Eeriva flat out told Yaniqui she wasn't going to be given any chores on the ship until her "mood improved," spurring a fight. Hloban caught Yaniqui and Waquas make eye contact and glance hastily away from each other. The only person it seemed Yaniqui didn't have a problem with was Keyad. No surprise there as Keyad had the most calming personality on the *Caneille*. They talked haltingly about Wea Saa as Keyad set dry beans to soak.

Finally, it was time for Hloban to go to sleep. The dorm was blissfully dark and soundproof. He quickly stripped to his underwear and climbed into bed before anything else could happen and promptly went to sleep comfortably for the first time since Akar Evion.

He was having the most wonderful dream—of what, he wasn't sure, all he knew was his dick was pulsing pleasantly—when suddenly all traces of sleep were gone and replaced with something so alert, he wondered if he was having a heart attack.

He frantically brought forth thoughts of Loera, but those thoughts drained away as quickly as they came. His body curved toward her on its own.

Yaniqui pressed herself close to his side and ran her bottom lip down his shoulder. One of her hands sank down his chest and he felt a leg slide on top of his, slightly chillier than his own sleep-drenched body.

Hloban wondered if he could enjoy something if he knew it was terribly wrong and his brain screamed against it the entire time, blocking out any pleasurable sensations with a message of doom.

It turned out he could.

Her lips made their way up to his stubble and found his ear. She took a delicate nip of the flesh under his lobe and whispered, "You can touch me too, you know."

"Yaniqui, we can't," he tried to keep his voice quiet. Any member of the crew could come into the dormitory and find them any moment. And, honestly, everyone had to know Hloban and Yaniqui were in there together. The craft was so small everyone was naturally tuned in to each other's positioning. "It's not supposed to be this way," he insisted.

It took every ounce of strength he had to push away from her. He collected her hands and held them tightly between his. Hloban groaned slightly in his throat. How many times had he wondered what his perfect life was supposed to be like? If the woman that was supposed to be his would have felt any different than the woman he ended up with? Since Akar had released the photos of her, he had thought about pressing her body onto his more than once. Just the two of them, alone. Except they weren't alone. He wasn't stopping because he was a good guy. He was stopping because they were going to get caught...and also it was wrong.

"Hloban." No one could say his name like her. He heard her swallow. "You put aside *everything* to rescue me. Who else would you have done that for?" She leaned against him and brushed her cheek against his neck.

There was a brief thought of stopping her but the logic washed away.

"We're supposed to be together. I've waited years to be with you. You've sacrificed so much. There are things you deserve. Wouldn't that make things better?"

Hloban's fingers flexed and pulled her closer, kneading her warm skin. He couldn't help it. This was supposed to be his. He was entitled to it.

"Just a little," Yaniqui murmured. "There's nothing wrong with that."

For someone who occupied so many of his thoughts in so many ways, her body was unfamiliar. He felt guilty of more betrayal as he noticed Yaniqui's stomach wasn't dappled by stretchmarks or age. He breathed in the scent of her clean hair.

Hloban was supposed to spend his life with this woman. Sleep in the same bed. Have children together. She was the predetermined best match for him. Hloban traced a hand upward, cupping the bottom of a breast, and put his lips against her shoulder.

This was all. It was all he'd ever have with her. He'd done wrong, but maybe this memory of something so complete, so perfect and predestined, would allow him to move on. He should have had so much with Yaniqui. But he had made a choice.

He pulled his hands back. "Yaniqui." Her name hung in the air. "I can't. I really can't."

A shaky breath. "You don't love me?"

Hloban's eyes darted away, guilty. "Of course, I love you. But we can't be together." He sat and pulled the covers up prudishly.

"But can't you see what's wrong with that?"

Hloban gave a deep sigh. He was terrified, but also immensely grateful no one had yet come into the dormitory. He swung his legs over the side of the bunk.

"Yaniqui, I don't know why any of this happened. I always expected to spend my life with you. Then the solar flare...I thought you were dead. I kept searching, kept looking out for any surviving Wea Saavian, but I never expected to find anyone, much less you. Searching became a ritual. It was a way to remind myself of how much

I'd lost, how it was okay that Earth didn't feel like home because it wasn't. That it was okay that Loera and I had differences because we *were* different.

"And then we found you. I know this has been hard, but I'm not sorry we came for you. Even if you and I can't be together—in that way—I wanted to make you safe. And you deserve so much more than what I can give to you. Things just didn't go right. I have a whole family and life waiting for me on Earth."

The room went still and Hloban desperately wished he could see her face.

"What does that mean for me?"

"I don't know, Yani." He was quiet while he thought how best to say it. "But the best part is you can build something for yourself too. And when it comes down to it, I don't think you really love more than the idea of me."

Yaniqui shivered but not from the cold. Her voice was raw. "My whole life has been about loving you."

"And now it's going to be about so much more than that."

She let a deep breath out in a crashing wave. "I do love you though. But I can also see that this isn't what you want. I don't crisping understand it at all, but okay, I won't try anymore."

"Thank you," Hloban said in relief. "You will always be my family. I will help you build a new life and there will be a day when you're infinitely happier than you ever expected. In the meantime—"

She nodded and finished his sentence, wholeheartedly disheartened. "Boundaries."

Hloban stood and she curled up in the bed. He could hear her sniff back tears. He was crying too though she couldn't see it in the darkness. He reached out a hand for her.

"For me too, please," she said. "I'd like to be alone."

# Chapter 25

Ippa
Jupiter Station

Ippa's bunk was simple. A thin white blanket and small white neck roll topped it and space underneath stowed her regulation-sized bags neatly. It was a shared space with eighteen other women along with a few children traveling to Earth. Ippa didn't expect to share a space with the workers—she hadn't on the transverser—and now worried that her lack of friendliness on the craft was a mistake.

She spent the first few days filling out paperwork and stopped in the medical bay to give a blood sample. A giant sign on the wall warned against blood samples for cold-blooded creatures as well as those with nonregenerating bodies, unlike her own.

Ippa walked the halls of the Jupiter Station looking for the office of the transitional counselor. The station was one giant, slow-turning ring with huge windows along the outer perimeter that gave view to Jupiter's raging storms. The station's gravity was ever-stable and slightly more intense than on the transverser, but Ippa thought she adapted well enough. Medical and psychiatric testing were going well and nearly completed, but Ippa's most important stage on the Jupiter

Station was yet to begin.

Though Ippa was out there—in the far reaches of rural, backwater space, on the verge of doing real, original research—she felt every movement shadowed. Or utterly not shadowed rather, for it was approval that Ippa wished for most. After years in the rigid education system, Ippa was used to knowing every step was the right one to take, every advancement would bring her closer to her ultimate goal of graduating with highest honors. Someone was always there to tell her if she was doing a good job or not.

Now, as a regular adult in the galaxy doing her own thing, Ippa couldn't be certain of anything.

The hall split off and finally there was a sign. Ippa went right and located the transitional counseling office. The open door revealed a tiny room. She smoothed her tunic before peeking in to find an Earthling woman with four bunches of tight curls on the back of her head that looked like they had almost been whipped, pinned, and sprayed into shape but, once the woman turned away from her mirror, had revolted against her.

"Hello," the Earth lady said, peering briefly up through her lashes, "give me one second." She returned to her work. The woman took up most of the space in her office-like closet.

"Not a problem Mrs. Potscha"—there was a small name plate on the desk—"take all the time you need."

Ippa busied herself with reading a poster about the process. The posters alone on the station were fascinating. It would be a lot easier for everyone if a station attendant announced all the information once during arrival. Instead, there were posters everywhere with directions, colloquial sayings, and important information accompanied by pictures of Earth animals in funny poses.

The woman nodded to herself at the end of her task and said, "All right, come in. You're the student, correct?"

"Yes, Mrs. Potscha." Ippa sat when she gestured to the tiny chair opposite her. The gesture brought about the start of the interview and Ippa felt instantly more comfortable. How many interviews and presentations had she done in her lifetime? If one imagined the real world was school, maybe one *could* get through the mess of adulthood.

Mrs. Potscha found Ippa's file on her tablet and skimmed it.

"You're here as part of the Windfall Program, is that right?"

"Windfall? I am not sure the program—"

"Oh, it's known as the Educative Experience Program throughout the galaxy. The Windfall Program is our nickname, an inside joke." She cleared her throat primly. "What will you study?"

"Well, the biblioplaza of Shou University is strong on language, geography, and general Earth culture, but I'm particularly interested in how Earth has changed since Contact was made. Earth is still within a few generations of original Contact, so it'd make a great case study on the topic. I'd also like to make some general explorations so we can update our sources and take some biological and geologic samples, within reason and with permission, of course." Ippa smiled. She nailed it. She should have, after all the money her parents invested in interview coaches.

"Mmm-hmm, and this would all be to update the records at Shou University?"

Ippa improvised. "I want to keep my options open. I might write the study on Earth under my name, instead of the university's. It depends on where my research takes me."

Mrs. Potscha nodded. "I read through your proposal. Everything seems to be in order as far as the content. Earth isn't able to dictate the subject matter, regardless. I will give you the forms for any organic samples you wish to take. You must submit the form for approval *before* taking the samples, even if the organic owner is willing."

Ippa confirmed that she understood and brightened with anticipation of the end.

"What's left is a matter of your educative sponsor."

Ah, everything else was a precursor. This was the real dish.

"You listed Shou University on your paperwork...but when I contacted them for your records," Mrs. Potscha said dryly, "they claimed you had been expelled. How do you explain that discrepancy?" The woman looked down and typed something while waiting for an answer.

*Oh crisping papers.* Ippa did not expect a far and away place like this to have access to Shou student records.

"Really. What? Are you sure?" was all Ippa could come up with.

The woman kept typing furiously.

"I mean, I knew I was on thin ice, as you Earthlings like to say, but I thought if I did a good job with this case study, I would be able to regain my place. I am an excellent researcher. I can share my latest papers to attest to my credibility—"

At that, the woman looked Ippa in the eye. "It's not a matter of your work, dear, but your *sponsor*. Without any overhead organization to vouch for you, you are simply not eligible for the program."

"I have a place set up to live. An Earthling named Loera Milson is going to let me stay with her. She runs an antimatter fuel lab and offered to create contacts for me in New Washington."

Ippa sensed the woman pause and reassess. "Yes, I know Loera Milson," Mrs. Potscha said. "Or I know *of* her."

Ippa held her breath.

"Loera is a very good connection for you to have. Mmm, it sounds like a good plan." Mrs. Potscha stared down at her tablet. "But, alas, I regret to inform you I just cannot break the regulations on this."

Ippa struggled to keep her breath. She looked at the woman's messy shelves stacked with thick binders and the room felt all too small. The mess of it veered close as her perspective warped. She exhaled strongly through her nose.

"I see," Ippa said, though she did not. "I apologize for the discrepancy with the paperwork. But surely there's some arrangement we can come to. I did study at Shou University. I—"

Mrs. Potscha leaned forward and rested her heavy bosom on her desk. "It's not a matter of what arrangement you and I can come to. When we take on a scholar, Earth incurs many expenses to transport and assist them in exchange for the opportunity for one of our own students to travel to an alien planet, um, alien to us that is, and perform research. We would like nothing more than to connect one of ours with that opportunity. However, without a recognized placement within a university, your presence on Earth would not count toward the program. Earth would get nothing from the arrangement."

"But I came all this way." Ippa was embarrassed to hear the whine in her voice.

Mrs. Potscha sighed. "Dear, you should have confirmed all of your paperwork with your educative organization before setting out on an interstellar expedition." She gestured meaningfully at the poster *Tips to Know Before Traveling to Earth.*

"Does Earth have any other visitor programs?" Ippa asked, feeling small.

"Earth has unfortunately not been cleared by the Joint Council for tourism at this time. Our labor program, refugee resettlement, and the Educative Experience Program are the only opportunities for individuals to visit or live on Earth.

"You do not qualify as a refugee. Ergo, you have three options. Find another educative organization to sponsor you, apply to the labor program, or take the next flight off the Jupiter Station. If you choose this last option, you will have to pay us back for room and board."

"When will the next transverser depart?" Ippa asked in a small voice.

"Forty-three rotations."

Ippa walked down the hallway dazed. She was supposed to be a magnificent whiz kid. Scratch that. She *was* a magnificent whiz kid. How could she have gotten herself stuck on the edge of the galaxy with no funds and no plan? Her parents could likely scramble to get together enough funds to cover the cost of traveling back home, but the expense of staying on a transitional station for forty-three rotations would be enormous. Calculations broke out in her mind, but she pushed them aside. If she went that route, it'd bankrupt the family, and she'd come home a fool as well as a failure. That option was clearly, and most definitely, out.

Ippa scanned her temporary pass and the pocket door slid open. The rest of the room was blocked from others who might be in the hallway, so Ippa skirted around the partition in a huff, went immediately to her bunk, and screeched into her thin pillow.

Really, what did Ippa know about Earth? The highest geographical point? That their dinosaurs went extinct before they could evolve intelligent brains? That they ate popped corn?

"Girl, what's got you?"

Ippa bolted up right. Most of the bunks were empty, but three women were congregated together close by. They watched Ippa with distanced amusement.

"Sorry. Just a rough day."

"Hey, I know you," a tiny woman with sleek hair down to her wide hips said. "You're that computer lady."

Her friend snapped her fingers. "Yeah. You didn't bunk with us on the ride over, why're you here now?"

Ippa sat up and smoothed back her short hair. The pillow had made it go frizzy.

"I was in a contributor role on the transverser. Here, I'm trying to find a way to Earth."

The tiny woman squinted her eyes as if Ippa's story would open unto her. "You don't look like a refugee with that blue hair."

"It's my natural color," Ippa snapped.

"Sorry, sweetie. You in the labor program?"

Ippa worked incredibly, incredibly hard to keep judgment out of her voice. "No, I'm not in the labor program." It didn't work.

The third woman let out a low "ooohh," and they all looked at each other.

"Blue thinks she's better than us."

"No!" Crisps, Ippa was breaking all the rules of Cultural Anthropology 101. "Of course not. I'm upset because I was supposed to go to Earth to study it—do a research project—and my university won't sponsor me."

"Why's that?"

"I was expelled."

All three broke out laughing. When the woman who let out the "ooohh" saw Ippa's expression, she waved her hand. "Don't worry about it so much. I was kicked out of my university too. I was going to be a fashion designer. But, tuition, you know?"

Ippa forced herself to breathe. "Oh, I'm sorry to hear that." She found herself telling the other women about her failures.

"You didn't fail," Tiny—who was named Kim—said. "It sounds terrible."

That earned only a shrug from Ippa. "I'm trying to think what other educative organization I could contact and get approval from."

Nothing on her home planet was registered in the program. That was one of the points she made to convince her parents to let her go to The Shou—the expanded opportunities.

Another woman walked in and Kim and the other two lost interest. They gathered around the newcomer and asked how her interview went. It was clear they all knew each other from the long journey to the Sol System.

Could Ippa truly put herself in their place? Take part in the same lifestyle? All of that energy spent trying to be the best in her star system, getting into Shou University and investing years of her life…all to become a migrant laborer on Earth?

Ippa knew the reality. Any well-educated person did. You needed to move locations because of war or medical accessibility, or because you dared hope for a life where gang violence didn't threaten your children. Someone said they would help you out, but along the way you racked up debts and got pushed into meager living conditions. Your original dreams are gone and all that's left is to try to work to free yourself and get back to where you started. Worst-case scenario, you are bodily taken and harvested for biological material.

Ippa believed in Pleplo's Principle of Available Decision Making. No other door stood open to Ippa.

She stood and went to find a poster about the labor program.

# Chapter 26

D-68
The Catchment, Earth

When D-68 comes to the surface again, he does not know how far away the human compound is. The one with iron bars that bite with the power of lightning and the hairy beast that helped him. The experience is fading, but the words he learned remain. He dug to the surface because he was in desperate need of sustenance. There were no crunchy roots in these caves and barely any trickles of water, remnants of the gushing waterways of old that originally formed them.

D-68 leaves the hole by dark.

Ahead of him is a vast forest of Earth trees. Instead of venturing out, he goes up. D-68 climbs the tiny cliff face easily. It would have been training grounds for the kits on his planet. Still, he is more comfortable on rock than the soft ground.

The planet stinks. Outside the rocky tunnels, his breaths come wet. Tiny pollen spores irritate his sensitive nasal pads. He wants a sniff of air that is arid and does not take one by the nose. For all his hate of the wet air, he wants something thick and juicy to crush between his teeth. He eventually climbs down and crosses the ground like the Earth beasts. There is mud and D-68 does not like how it squishes between his platelets and stays there. The food he forages is limp and barely chewable. Pitiful leaves come off the tall, brittle trees.

A female human walks underneath. It is the first human he's been close to since he escaped and he is revolted. He forgot how small they are. How very many scents come off their body. D-68 considers dropping down on it and destroying the creature.

But he cannot justify extinction of something simply for his rage. Eating meat was a foreign idea to him until he was taken captive, and still, the idea disgusts him. Unless he is formally at war with another clan, he will not kill.

He looks up at the pale orb hanging in the sky, and beyond to the fragments of light scattered across the great abyss. D-68 never thought about what was up in the stars, but now that he knows, he cannot shake it. Sitting by himself, hidden in the hole, he thought and remembered things that were buried far down in his cranium. D-68 knows that even if he goes back to his home, he will be different. His hamlet is at the very bottom and when you go up, up, up, you come to the place where things are ugly and wet and every being hates others.

By necessity, he finds two water sources. The first is a big water, bigger and more ferocious than he ever thought water could be. He hears echoes of a settlement close by, but he is so thirsty he chances exposure to draw a drink. It tastes like death and he knows he will not go there again. In the forest, D-68 finds a small stream. He drinks heavily to fill his stomachs. There along the banks, he finds thin, wet plants to eat. They catch in his broad teeth, but there is nothing better.

He sleeps by day in the hole and comes out the next night. D-68 eats tiny colored buds off the plants. Later, his waste turns watery and burns its way out, dripping below to the ground. Sickness and weakness overtake him. The biome is not enough to sustain one such as him. He knows not what he can do to save himself, but action is the only way forward. To stay in hiding would be to starve and die.

So, it is with purpose that D-68 walks toward the settlement. He cannot call it a hamlet. Their smells waft through the air. He watches several long stretches and sees lights glinting in the darkness. These dirty humans live so close they breathe their night air on each other.

He circles the perimeter laboriously over several nights. He is not interested in the humanoids, but he sees and smells things that are not human. They are not of his kind, but all manners of creatures, some big like him, others small. He smells a sordid sweat, the sickly sweet smell of plant foods, rot, and crushed rock.

Finally, with the orb gone from the sky, D-68 approaches as carefully as he can under the cover of absolute darkness. He walks a path between nests and homes. He hears voices and smells food. A kit mewls nearby.

A skeletal-looking creature beckons to him from the darkness. It stands from a nighttime perch and utters a strange occurrence of sounds. D-68 snorts. He tries his own language. The creature looks away disinterestedly.

"Speak us," D-68 says in the sounds of the captors.

"Yes, I speak their language," the other croaks. "Unfortunate that we have to bring ourselves down to their level to communicate. Where are you from, friend?"

"Down."

"Under the crust of their planet?"

D-68 does not know what else to say. What to ask. What to tell. He feels foolish.

"No, I think you are from the stars, like me." It points up at the black and stumbles upon what confuses D-68 most, of all of this. The black looks similar to the night sky from his planet but a different pattern. D-68 went up into them, but how are the stars also up here?

The other creature takes no notice of his inner musings. "Friend, are you new to this place?"

D-68 takes this small opening, "New me."

"First things first, as the Earthlings like to say."

"Earthling."

"The creatures that currently rule this planet. First things first. Are you in need of shelter? Sustenance?"

"Need, need me."

"I'm going to take you to someone who can help you. Follow me, friend."

The unlikely pair sets off. Their short walk is the first meeting between their two species in the history of the universe. It is not due to diplomacy, exploration, or trade. It comes from displacement and a will to survive.

They arrive at a low structure.

"Wait here."

D-68 stands in the dark, under the stars, unsure of everything.

A spindly-looking creature with many legs comes out. The thin, wiry limbs glisten in the moonlight. It stops and assesses D-68 much like how he assessed Jeb long ago.

D-68 is the superior in size and strength, but he feels a power and rage emitting from the animal. It is a rage he can respect. If it were humanoid, directing that animosity in his direction, D-68 would crush it gladly. But it is an animoid. And if it has anger, on this planet, D-68 is sure they are comrades. Same enemy. Same goals.

It opens its mouth and issues a *tsk*, translated by a human boy, who stands behind. "He says he can help you. But he needs something from you in exchange."

"Hey, you gotzz a light?" one of the other animoids asks as they stand under the trees. D-68 shakes his head. He would rather use their gestures than speak their words to communicate.

A second creature stands, reaches inside his jacket the color of the spongy moss that grows in the caves north of D-68's hamlet, and throws a fire starter to the other. The first lights the roll and a cloying sweet scent permeates the air. It's the same smell that often comes from the containers he moves in exchange for food. Leggs offered D-68 the same thing multiple times, but the scent revolts him. The smoke makes one slow. He also refused shelter. He would much rather hang on the tiny cliffs or burrow underneath the ground than sleep in the night air of so many from so many worlds.

"I'm 'vo," the one with the fire says.

D-68 looks him over again. He has a fleshy stomach like the humans—what a weakness to have—and a broad nose. His skin flakes along one side of his neck.

"How long have you been on-planet?"

The one smoking growls like an animal. "Izz don't remember any other place. Izz don't think Izz was born here though. I've been working for Leggzz for a while."

D-68 speaks, "Come you?"

"Whatz that, ugly? You're gonna have to learn to talk better if yer going to zsurvive here."

'vo says, "Yes, perhaps he should take lessons from you. You're practically a native."

The tiny one with the thick voice and short stature scowls, but 'vo continues, "I was born on a transverser. A huge one, always breaking down in the middle of nowhere. My mother—I didn't know my father—my mother looked after the livestock, most to be transported, some to be eaten on the craft."

The short one looks disgusted. "What sortz of beasts did you transport to eat? Waz they Intelligent?"

"Once I did see a proper animoid in among them. He asked me for water. I was taken, or sold perhaps, from my mother. I woke up in the bowels of a different spacecraft in a pain I've never experienced before or since." 'vo points to a faded but knotty scar just above the human trousers he wears. "I still don't know what I'm missing, but I keep living so it must not have been that important. I was sold from here to there and then finally rescued by a police craft and sent here. This place isn't too bad. It's the first planet I set foot on."

A dim red light shines on them from above and they back up to watch a minicraft land in the clearing. Unlike the roaring engines of the craft D-68 was taken to Earth on, this one is silent. Behind D-68 and the others are stacks of crates they brought from a location outside the settlement.

This is not the first time D-68 has been to the clearing. The first time, he hauled crates from an underground space in the settlement to the forest where they loaded them on a spacecraft. He has gained some of his strength back after his confinement, but even so, it took many trips to bring all of the items. D-68 never saw inside them, but he could sense Earth rock and smelled dried Earth plants and the sweet, unnatural smell that makes his head wave and ache. The first experience stands out in D-68's weak memory. The others have already faded. D-68 knows this is one of the things he does for the many-legged one.

Tonight, D-68 is hungry. He has been hungry since he was taken from his planet, but it grows in intensity. His stomach does not just crave food. His body has not replenished the minerals it needs for a very long time.

He distracts himself by carrying two crates. They are not heavy, but they are big and his leg is still prone to difficulty. Near the craft, he sets one package on the ground so he can carry the other through the small door. D-68 hardly fits. He pushes the crate in and against a wall. The Earth human who flew the craft to the clearing pulls strap after strap down from the ceiling, securing them into place. It is the same human every time and the only one that D-68 comes into contact with besides the boy translator. The Earthling hardly looks at D-68.

As if it doesn't see D-68 as a credible threat.

D-68 wonders if he could fly the craft himself. Each time he loads or unloads items, he studies what the human does. Already he has identified how to open the doors and thinks he could operate the talking piece of it, the radio, on his own. Late at night, the controls just a step away, the idea seems feasible. During the day, when he is in the rock cavern he scraped out, he knows it is useless. He will never be able to operate the craft.

If there is a chance he could do it himself, D-68 would do it now. But he knows there is none. His hands do not fit the controls. D-68 wonders about the others moving cargo with him. Are they trustworthy? Do they want to leave too?

He is tired of waiting. The many-legged one tells him he needs to be patient. He will get D-68 off-planet.

But what is the point? D-68 does not even know how to find his world. And what would he go back for? If his partner is alive, she is better off without him, weak and dumb as he is. He could not provide for the kits with his leg damaged. It is better for her to find a new mate.

And the Earthlings would not leave him alone. They are here and they are on his planet.

The three move the last of the boxes and the other two animoids start in the direction of the settlement. He will never sleep there. There is little protection among the weak structures. He turns, intending to head to the rocky outcrop and sleep.

Several nights later, D-68 goes to the meeting place. 'vo is there.

"Follow me, big guy." He smells sweet. "We've got a new assignment tonight."

"Speak you. Good."

'vo smiles. To D-68, he looks like an Earthling when he smiles. "My larynx is similar. I can make their words easily. Don't worry about it. I don't think Leggs wants you for your voice. Our shipment's live tonight."

"Food?" D-68 works hard to make the inflection with his voice and turn the Earth word into a question. He doesn't notice the change, but he now often holds two thoughts in his head at the same time. Regurgitating the word is exhausting work and he feels disgust at the thought of eating other living beings. How it must go down the throat hot and thick.

"Bodies. There's a lot of those here, in the Catchment. Bodies are wealth but not when they're not being used. Someone has to capitalize on it. That's us."

D-68 is wary. He does not want to come into contact with the humanoid side of the settlement, he thinks as he moves doggedly through the dark night. Disturbing Earthling affairs increases his chance of being found by the ones with the guns, the ones who took him.

He sees a pinprick of electric light before it disappears ahead of him.

"Now, what we need is young. Either young and strong, or young and beautiful. Either sold for fighting or fucking. That's what makes this universe go round. Unless you're going to eat them. And you and I eat cheaper than the likes of them," 'vo says, but D-68 hardly listens.

He is not concerned if the many-legged one takes Earthlings. The same was done to D-68. That is the way these species relate to each other. He is not obligated to protect any creature, though he knows his feelings are born from apathy.

If he did want to interfere though…D-68 decides not to pursue that course. He is big. He used to be a strong and skilled leader in his hamlet. But he has no power here. He cannot influence events around him. He can hardly protect himself. He needs food, much more food, so he must do what the many-legged one orders.

"Stand back there, D. That's right, in the shadows. You need to wait here," 'vo whispers.

They are on the outskirts of the settlement, the humanoid side. D-68 can smell the musky scent.

"Don't make any noise. I'll take care of everything. You're here for transport."

'vo walks away and D-68 waits a long time. He is hungry. The waiting gets dull, and then the waiting is full of anger as D-68 wonders if 'vo will return.

Finally, the smells around him grow stronger as humans come into distant view. Moist skin and breaths. It makes him sick.

'vo speaks to someone. "I don't dare carry this stuff around on me. Most people would just as soon steal from a guy like me as buy it."

A female voice speaks, "Girls, I don't think he has anything to sell us. I think he wants to have his way with us under the trees."

"Five of you and one of me, okay. But seriously, ladies, I'm a businessman. If you're going to get with this, I have to charge you."

Another voice, "Oh, and his own souteneur. If only girls could make double like a man."

The voices grow stronger as they get closer. D-68 thought 'vo looked like the humanoids and Earthlings, but now that he stands next to some, D-68 sees the difference. He wonders again what the fibers on their heads are for.

"Go ahead and try out a little before you purchase. My stuff is always the real deal. Just do me a favor and tell your friends, okay? Especially your beautiful friends."

'vo takes something from a box and prepares it. It's not sweet, but acidic. 'vo lights it and passes it quickly between the women. They stand talking and one of the women falls over.

There's laughter. "She's always the first to go," an Earthling says. Suddenly she sees that her other companions are on the ground too. A look of terror crosses her face and she spins and takes a step before she falls.

'vo ties their hands quickly with his own dexterous fingers.

"D, you're up. They'll be knocked out for a good long while. Take them to the pickup spot. I have to make sure there's no tracks."

D-68 snorts. He does not wish to touch their bodies. They disgust him. He also does not want to admit he is fearful. What if he breaks one open again?

The first body is warm. Brush and mud from the ground has seeped into its clothing. He slowly hoists one body across a shoulder and another on the other side. Perhaps he could take a third, but he is unused to the texture of their skin and decides two is enough.

There is a larger spacecraft in the clearing this time, one with two beings inside, the same human as before but also an animoid with a long neck. D-68 wonders why he takes such care with the bodies as he lowers them to the ground in front of the craft. It may be better for them to be dead than to waken.

He chastises himself. These are no more than animals. Their kind chatters so much, they must not have the brain power for complex thought like him. They live half-lives, unable to fully take in their surroundings. It makes no difference where they live those miserable lives out.

# Chapter 27

Lozen
The Catchment

A second bombing hit the original blocks, where the likes of Lin lived. For days, the ruins of the small building that served as a repair shop smoked, sketching wisps of ash across the sky that no one could ignore.

The Catchment was normally set on edge over supply shortages and territory disputes, but now it felt like it could boil over. It was scary wondering every time you visited a public space if it was about to blow up and end your life.

The bombing was the only event that could have taken the Catchment's mind off a group of young women that had disappeared. In the Catchment, people disappeared from time to time, but a whole group? Unless they all took off at the same time to try to escape into the capital—jumping the maze it was called—there weren't many other explanations with a happy ending.

Lozen wondered if or what the Karmas would do about it. She wasn't yet privy to their meetings, though she had spoken with Charla recently. When Lozen revealed she had identified who the bomber was, Charla was initially pleased. Lozen had made no mention of the GIA, making it sound like the discovery came from her time in the animoid blocks but felt like she had to warn Charla without giving anything away.

Lozen didn't relish the thought.

"You don't understand," Lozen told Charla. "He's not only big, he's strong." In the daylight on the shore where they met, Lozen could see the edges of a tattoo creeping out of Charla's low-necked collar, black on hickory brown.

"Lozen, we all play different parts on this team. Part of initiation is proving to us what you can do. Find where that nonperson sleeps and we'll take care of the rest," Charla said, her eyes probing Lozen.

She went on to make clear the next steps couldn't take as long for Lozen to complete. The invitation to join the Karmas would be revoked soon, unless she could provide the group with D-68's location.

It didn't go much better with Agent Tril when she checked in on the handheld the first time. Even worse the second. Tril insisted that they needed information soon. Not only where D-68 was staying, but who was helping him. For D-68 to do so much damage after arriving a short while ago, he clearly had a large network of other terrorists.

And then things got even worse when Monte came by the day before and discovered her friend was having second thoughts about everything.

It was time to get a handle on the situation. She wasn't leading an investigation—Lozen felt like she was being pulled around on one string before lurching in another direction. Charla, Agent Tril, Leggs, they all had their own agendas. It was time for Lozen to find out what those agendas were.

So, Lozen ordered a drink, more lighter fluid than fermented grain or fruit, she was sure. She brought the cup under her nose but didn't let it linger. It burned harshly. She turned and leaned casually against the dilapidated bar.

The Shirianhole was named for the burrow of an alien animal Lozen would never see. It was a dive bar in the animoid blocks. Every drinking establishment in the Catchment was a dive bar, but Lozen visited only the ones filled with bodies like hers.

She wasn't the only humanoid, but likely the only Earthling there. It was dark outside and dim inside. Two bare bulbs hung from the ceiling over the bar. There was a candle on one table. Languages, clicks, and coughs mixed throughout the room. The atmosphere felt like any humanoid bar. One group gambled in the corner, and two females—women?—dished to each other loudly, only whispering the name of the being they were talking about.

Something hopped up on the bar next to Lozen. She startled but quickly relaxed. It was nice to see a familiar furry blue face.

"Thought I might see you here someday."

"Well, you know more than me, then." Lozen reached out tentatively, asking permission, and the creature pressed the back of its neck into her hand. She scratched gently.

"What are you anyway?"

"A minkin. Much better looking than a shirian, I can assure you. Are you going to drink that?"

"I think I'd die." Lozen set the cup on the bar and turned back to the scene while the minkin lapped at the drink.

"That's your mark," he whispered. "Go."

Lozen fought to wipe the surprise from her face. She stretched casually to turn and watch as an alien left the bar.

The minkin rolled his eyes. "Go."

Lozen went, no questions asked. She wondered at the wisdom of it but there wasn't time. Besides, she'd never got any feelings of animosity from the minkin before. She left the humid warmth of the Shirianhole and went out into the cool night. The rains had finally taken a break and the mud had dried up. Lozen walked carelessly, even overtaking the tall slender alien, naked but for pants, and purposefully darted into another pathway. Mindful of getting lost in the animoid blocks in the dark, she waited for him to pass, then peered around the corner and followed at a careful distance. She swallowed when he slid through a crack in the fencing. The forest.

It'd be easier to follow him there, but lately there was something about the limitless maze that made Lozen nervous. With Charla's disappointed face on her mind, she slipped in a few moments after the animoid. She paused in the shadow of the wall and listened intently. Then, Lozen followed, able to keep tabs on the sound of the alien's clumsy walking.

Eventually, they came to a clearing. Lozen kept well outside the moonlight. The alien joined another that sat on a pile of barrels and a few crates. A form emerged from the trees, directly opposite Lozen. Even at that distance, her heart stopped. He was huge. Seeing D-68 felt akin to sighting a bear in the woods.

He set down two barrels.

The alien Lozen had followed dumped out a bag in front of D-68 who gestured angrily to the pile of leaves. Muted conversation drifted over. "Take it up with Leggs." He said something more about food and the voices dropped to a murmur.

A ship appeared silently overhead and lit the clearing with soft red light. A rabbit in the thicket next to Lozen startled and raced away. Lozen's stomach plummeted as D-68's attention was pulled from his food. He looked intently in her direction and put his head up into the air, as if he was sensing something.

*Oh fuck.*

Her scent!

Lozen shrank farther into the tendrils of the brush, heart galloping wildly.

D-68 seemed satisfied and began loading the items into the ship with the others. She realized the wind ran parallel to them both. That wasn't a mistake she'd make again.

Lozen crept backward as silently as she could. She'd complete her heart attack in the privacy of her own shack.

A welcome patch of sunlight warmed Lozen's skin as a nearly silent ship shimmered as it landed, near invisible. Lozen waited in the trees until Agent Tril stepped out of the cruiser. She beckoned Lozen forward.

Lozen advanced eagerly despite her distrust of Tril. "This is amazing. How does it do that?" Lozen immediately wanted to retract her unsophisticated question.

Tril didn't seem to mind. "This ship reflects light, like a mirror, but it can blend that light into the colors around it, the ones your eye expects to see, rather than simply bouncing the light back. The surface is more similar to thousands of prisms than a mirror."

"A prism?"

"It's a glass triangle that refracts light as it travels through. The light is bent not bounced. They're smart prisms that control the speed at which different colors travel through to match its surroundings. Would you like to ride in it?"

"Yes!" Even if D-68 was never captured, riding in the ship would be worth all of the trouble and risk. Lozen climbed in and took her time looking at the control panel. Tril explained the buttons and screens in fair detail and showed Lozen how to strap in. The Catchment felt far away for the first time in Lozen's life.

The ship barely rumbled as it lit up. She sensed the landing gear leave the ground. Lozen watched the outside carefully through the windshield, her mouth open. Quicker than she expected, they took off up into the sky. The trees grew smaller and Lozen spotted a jut of rock from the cliff line. Then the edge of the Catchment appeared. It was all laid out before her. She gasped. The Catchment was huge. There was the lake far in the distance, the road system opposite, and a greening forest all around.

"Where are we going?"

"I have a surprise for you and then I'm taking you into our offices."

Soon, a highway with speeding cars stretched out underneath them. The space elevator twinkled faraway on the horizon. Then there were homes, huge houses fifty humanoids could live in and each building had large squares of green grass. Lozen saw a black dog chase a ball, bigger than any dog to be found in the Catchment.

"Are these all Earthlings who live here?"

"For the most part, yes. The capital is about 95 percent Earthling and 5 percent alien. It's the highest density of aliens in the world after the labor camps and the Catchment."

"Are the aliens just humanoid or are there animoids too?"

"Just a few."

Lozen was studying a blue rectangle below them and realized it was a swimming pool. Lozen wondered what it would be like to have your own lake, one you could make sure was always healthy enough, always clean enough.

Agent Tril touched down in a cruiser parking lot. She then gave Lozen a small stack of clothes and told her to put it on in the bath capsule. Inside, Lozen pulled on a silky smooth blouse with tiny buttons along the shoulder seam and pants that showed off her shapely legs. Lozen hadn't bathed for three days, but the new clothes made her feel cleaner than ever before in her life.

It was time to clarify exactly what this was. "You want to show me what I can have if I help you catch D-68?"

"You can live on this side of the wall. You will work, but it will be easier. You will have access to hospitals and get your surgery. If you have children, they'll go to school and get good jobs."

Lozen was quiet. She thought about Monte and Uzzie and the Karmas. All the people that would never have this.

"I think you have more information than you're telling us, Lozen. You're resistant, I can feel it. Do you feel bad for the animoid?"

Lozen shrugged, then said, "No, there's just a lot going on here and I want to sort everything out." She didn't speak aloud her worries that she was being manipulated in a situation she could not clarify.

"You're what we call a field information gatherer. I'm the expert. And it doesn't even end with me. When he's captured, D-68 will go in front of a judge and jury. He'll answer only for proven crimes. Remember, he was brought to Earth because he killed a human. He killed another when he escaped. And, yes, I'm fairly certain he is the bomber."

Tril sounded so assured of her place in the system. Her belief in the system.

They walked in silence to an open-air restaurant. It was completely unlike the small food stands in the Catchment. Lozen saw a woman her age with a baby in a sling and she wondered at how different her life would have been if she had been born a few miles over. Lozen sat in a plush chair while Tril ordered at the counter and eventually brought over two dishes.

"Have you had ice cream before?"

Lozen nodded, a little disappointed. She tried some as a girl with her aunt. It was a brittle, crystalized substance.

Lozen took her first bite. Saliva flooded her mouth as the sweetness hit her. She devoured the rest of the ice cream in silence, only pausing to open her mouth for more pieces of chocolate and candied strawberries.

What would Lozen tell Monte to do? To take it?

Yes. Yes, she would.

The GIA office building was easily the largest building Lozen had ever been in. It was an immense concrete behemoth dotted with tiny rectangular windows. Everything was smooth, neat, and professional. Humans buzzed in and out of the building like the colony it was.

At security, Agent Tril flashed her badge and was waved through, but Lozen had to write her name down on a screen. She wrote out the letters carefully, trying to look as if she did this every day. Then Lozen looked into an iris scanner and passed through a body sensor.

All these people a short ride from the Catchment lived an entirely different existence. They had clean clothes and professional jobs that required them to walk busily through wide, brightly lit hallways. Most of Lozen's days were filled with the small actions it took to secure food and water. There were odd jobs on her shack and now with the Karmas. No, Lozen didn't want to think of the Karmas. She'd figure things out later.

They passed the glass walls of a conference room. There was a long table with no middle, just a brief stretch of counter on the outside for the agents to hook their tablets into. Information displayed in the center. A group of workers took their seats and the windows frosted over for privacy.

Lozen and Tril found their own empty room and went inside. It smelled pleasant, yet bland. Tril activated a wall screen with a brief wave of her hand.

"You saw the holo of D-68, but you haven't seen him in action. I don't think you know how dangerous he is. This is a clip of him escaping last winter."

Lozen saw a grimy-looking building with a lacework of metal

covering the windows. Towers stood along the perimeter wall every two hundred yards.

"What is this?"

"It's the Animoid Detention Center." Tril zoomed in slightly. "It's less than ten miles from the Catchment. We passed it on the way here."

"But it didn't hold D-68."

"No. It didn't. Watch."

Even with all of the security around her, anxiety and fear crawled up her throat as she took in once more the huge, powerful arms with great talons on the end. If there was ever a poster child for interstellar crime, he was it. Lozen's arms prickled when she thought of watching him through the trees just a few nights ago, and at the thought of what could have happened had the wind been blowing a different direction.

On the screen, D-68 grabbed a gun and threw it at a guard. It wasn't even a throw. It was like he shot the gun, the entire gun, no need for bullets, and it flew straight into the guard's gut. His otherworldly gait took him to the rock wall that he scaled almost elegantly. He disappeared over the side. The camera angle couldn't take the rest in.

"Did other cameras pick him up? Satellite?" Lozen asked.

"He would have been recaptured almost immediately, but he disappeared underground. The guards were utterly unprepared for that occurrence. I have one more video to show you." It was a quick clip, less than twelve seconds. D-68 was behind bars when he thrust his arm through a human and bellowed.

Lozen paled at how puny the human looked next to D-68. At how quickly he wiped out the man's life.

Through their own glass window, Lozen saw Agent Velazquez coming their way. He winked at Lozen when he saw her watching him.

"Remember, Lozen, you don't need to, and in fact shouldn't, approach him. We need to know where he's staying, where he regularly goes, and if there's anything that can link him to the bombing," Tril said.

Lozen felt heat rush to her ears. If she told them about the clearing, all of it would be over. She'd have a new life. A dangerous animoid would be apprehended.

But she'd lose Monte. The Karmas and the entire Catchment would hate her for working with the GIA. Should she give the information to Charla instead?

Velazquez walked in as Lozen asked, stalling for time, "Why was D-68 in a cage in that last clip? Why did he kill that person?"

"Who can say, Lozen? Sometimes these animals act out until they figure out who's in charge," Velazquez said.

Tril started up the video again. "One more to play."

It was drone footage from over the Catchment. The rusted, holey roofs were unmistakable. The creatures on the ground were visible only by the tops of their head, and Lozen belatedly recognized herself following a young boy. She watched herself reach up under her hairline and scratch at her bald stripe.

Her scalp burned and begged to be itched in real time, but Lozen stared intently at the screen, willing the sensation away.

"You followed me?" She wondered if the situation could get any more real.

"Part of it was for your safety, Lozen. And yes, we are committed to finding this murderer so we've followed you on several different occasions."

On-screen, Lozen and the boy ducked inside a low shelter.

Tril prompted, "Lozen, I want to help you. If you give me information about D-68, I can find you a new home. Change your life. Who did you go talk to?"

"His name was Leggs."

"Did he have information about D-68?"

"He said he had heard of him and that he'd try to learn more by the next time I returned."

Tril pulled up a GIA file filter. "What did he look like?"

"Long. Buggy. Didn't speak English. He had, like, a million legs."

Tril selected a box reading "more than ten limbs" and the only result that came up was the centipede.

"That's him."

Tril wrinkled her nose, and read aloud, "On Earth for twelve years. Transported here as a part of the extreme refugee resettlement program. Unqualified for labor camps. Endangered species."

"I know him now," Velazquez said. "He's working with another team on something. He wouldn't be caught up in this."

Tril looked at her partner with surprise. "There's no notes in his file."

"It's off the record. I only know because Burns asked my opinion—he was a potential perp on another case—and we both were surprised to learn he's a very low-level informant. Not a very good one, I gather. It was a dead end."

"No," said Lozen. Her voice grew more confident. "Leggs is trouble. The other animoids act like he's this huge boss. He gives me the creeps. It's not just how he looks. When he speaks—well, when the kid translates for him—you can tell he's used to getting what he wants."

It was all so much bigger than her. Lozen decided to tell the agents everything, including seeing D-68 in the forest. The only thing she held back was the Karmas.

"Leggs told me he'll tell me where D-68 is if he can secure placement in the capital. Like my deal."

Tril and Velazquez were silent.

"I can tell you, definitively, he'll never make it to the capital," Tril started.

"Isn't that speciesism?"

"No," said Velazquez, "it's just a fact."

"We'll have to vet this carefully and get some evidence," Tril said, sitting down in thought.

"But here's the thing, I think D-68 is working for Leggs in some capacity. Why would he sell out D-68 to you guys?"

"Betrayals in these instances aren't unheard of, but if that's what gets us D-68, fine," Tril said. "Lozen, you need to promise Leggs whatever he wants if he can give us the location of D-68, to be paid after capture."

"You want me to lie to him? What about me?" Lozen squeaked.

"By the time he finds out, you'll be in the capital. You'll never see him again."

# Chapter 28
### Yaniqui
### In Transit

The air lock door between Yaniqui and space—the one Yaniqui had first entered to find her long-lost love—was the only place she was hanging out these days. Actually, there were two doors. There was always two of everything between people and the cold darkness of space, except for that time Yaniqui was slowly going into hibernation with a dragon, wasn't that a laugh?

She put down the book Waquas lent her, leaned back on the door, and closed her eyes. The hum of machinery reminded her of the distant buzzing of beetle colonies on 4,278. Even with her eyes closed, it wasn't nearly hot enough and the air around her tasted stale in her mouth. Her hair was grimy in a way it never was on-planet and definitely not while with Akar.

Eeriva put her foot down about the daily showers. Yaniqui did the math…her water ration on board the *Caneille* was one-ninth what she was allotted in Akar's facilities. Maemi would have done the calculation quicker. Yaniqui's heart couldn't stop breaking. And no one else made it any easier for her.

"The system is maxed out at six people," Eeriva had pointed out to Keyad and Waquas, in front of Yaniqui.

Hloban had been sleeping, Yaniqui's thoughts were partly in the dark room with him (she promised to give him space but not to stop pining over him) so she hadn't been paying attention to the executive officer's discussions.

"Something we knew when we left Earth with six people on board, expecting a seventh," Waquas replied.

Eeriva smoothed back her hair. It was greasy too. "Yes, but we're not giving the systems keeping us alive enough support. I had expected to do three pit stops—we did one rushed stop that barely replenished our water system."

Yaniqui interrupted, "What did you say, Waquas? You left with an extra being who's no longer on board?"

She felt more than saw Eeriva grimace at what she considered Yaniqui's political correctness. To Eeriva, "being" was something she did, not a name to encompass the lives of others different than her.

"Patrick was captain when we left Earth. He died en route."

"He was very elderly," Keyad added.

"Oh, I'm sorry," Yaniqui said. "I had no idea."

And Yaniqui *was* sorry. Sorry someone had died coming to save her. Sorry there wasn't enough washing water and Eeriva was on edge about supplies. Sorry Adam wouldn't share his video games with her because she cracked the VR headset on her first time. (She was confused. She tried to jump the same time the spacecraft lurched and came down hard on her face.) Sorry she wasn't as young or kind or beautiful or worthy as they had all expected. Sorry Hloban was in love with someone else and she had no future with him.

Sorry most of all for Maemi.

Maybe that was why she had a sudden deep desire to be back on 4,278, before her identity was discovered. If things hadn't been perfect, at least she and Maemi had been together.

Yaniqui had tried talking the others into finding Maemi. It wasn't that they weren't willing. After their doomed rescue of her coming off better than they had hoped, they were eager even. When Yaniqui first came on board, there was a buzz of purpose as everyone talked and thought about where Maemi could be, skipping the sleep schedule entirely. Maybe Adam would have another brilliant idea. Keyad especially worked hard scouring the Wave and dark net for any clue or sign of Maemi. Yaniqui gathered that he genuinely wanted all six Wea Saavians together, to provide safety to each other and reconstruct the home he lost long ago.

The problem wasn't lack of will but lack of lead. Yaniqui had been heavily advertised, but traces of Maemi disappeared the first day she was owned by Akar. Yaniqui was heartbroken to have no way to find Maemi, was heartbroken again by Hloban, and was generally weirded out by the entire sequence of events.

Consequently, Yaniqui was spending more and more time hunkered down the hall, away from the living quarters under the guise of wanting a quiet spot to read. She had read every physical book on board—she was starting the book from Waquas for the second time—but more and more she stared at the wall and thought about how fate had let her down.

A voice carried down the hall, a little more enunciated than usual. As it was Hloban's voice, her destined true love who had gallantly come to save her, her ears perked up. She couldn't hear who he was talking to and ran through the mental list. Eeriva and Adam were sleeping. Waquas had said he was going below to run diagnostics on a troublesome piece of equipment. Keyad was in the gym.

Hloban was talking to himself.

Curious what he might be saying, she left the book lying on the floor and crept on her toes down the hall. At the corner, she squatted and strained her ears.

"—and with the unpredictable schedule with the nanny, it's been hard."

Hloban said, "I'm sorry…can your mom?"

The woman murmured something back.

Yaniqui's eyes widened.

It was Loera! It had to be. It struck Yaniqui odd that she hadn't heard any calls to Loera when others came through with semiregularity. She even saw Waquas take a video call with someone who was keeping up his farm while he was away. Hloban must have been making calls to Loera while Yaniqui was sleeping. She and Adam had just traded sleep schedules. Adam wanted to be on the same schedule as Eeriva, hopelessly optimistic she'd let him do more on the craft, and Yaniqui was desperate to see a little less of the woman. Regardless, Adam should have asked Waquas to teach him—even Yaniqui knew that.

Everything widened into focus when Yaniqui heard mention of herself.

"Everything's going okay there though? The girl...she's not traumatized from being separated from her mom?"

"She's upset, of course. It's awful not knowing where Nica is. I remember meeting her for the first time. I was terrified, but she gave me this enormous flower from her garden. It was the size of a dinner plate," Hloban said. He sounded hesitant, as if he wasn't sure Loera wanted to hear those memories.

Her mother was a welcoming gardener who gave prized flowers to little boys? That wasn't Yaniqui's experience. Her heart clenched at the thought of how much Maemi had gone through and how much she must have changed...to protect her daughter.

Neither Hloban nor Loera had yet used Yaniqui's name. Yaniqui sighed softly. Of course, *she* barely liked thinking Loera's name, but no one around her was considerate enough to avoid mentioning the woman who had swiped her man. But Hloban would be considerate...to his wife.

Loera went on. "Her room is done. I've been trying to prepare Obani for the new change. Oh, and I assigned a few things to Mari. She wants to know what grade to enroll her in. Early high school? Or maybe a little earlier to make up for her lack of education?"

High school? Middle school? It was clear Hloban had not yet cleared up the mistake. How young did Loera think she was? She was of course a few years younger than Hloban, but Loera was talking as if she was a child....

It felt wrong—what kind of age gap did Loera think there was?—but also deliciously juicy. She couldn't wait to see the look on Loera's face when she realized the person she had agreed to house was not some kid vaguely aware of a cultural tie between her and the guy who had come to save her from the bad guys, but a fully grown adult in love with her husband.

Blood thrummed in her ears. Maybe she had agreed to keep her distance from Hloban, but she felt gratified to inflict at least a bit of uncertainty into Loera's life, someone Yaniqui had to dislike on principle. Yaniqui was relatively sure she was going to keep her word and avoid trying to ensnare Hloban, but that didn't mean she didn't want him and his wife to suffer, at least a little. To make it clear to them that they had made a big fat crisping mistake and to be around in case it broke them up.

She snapped out of her daydreams when she heard the urgency in Hloban's voice.

"I gotta go, Loera—another spacecraft just blipped on our screen." Hloban had barely hung up when the alarm sounded for an incoming transmission request.

Yaniqui heard a rustle from the dormitory and stood. She stepped around the corner, blank-faced. No, she had not overheard the wife of the man she loved call her a little girl.

Hloban waved at her frantically and pointed to the dormitory. She could already hear Waquas replacing metal panels, the whirl of the hand tool coming from far below.

One ear on the console, Yaniqui strode purposefully, opened the door, and turned on the light in the dorm. She was already halfway to Hloban's side by the time she heard Adam stir and weakly protest the brilliant illumination in the middle of his REM cycle.

The *Caneille* slowed.

Yaniqui moved to Hloban's side. She looked at his strained face and gave a soft smile. She could do this. She could be his partner. Let him see she was there for him, always would be. In case an opportunity opened.

A raspy voice pulled through the vast gaping yawn of space.

"This is Captain Jung of *Transverser A00529*, identify yourself."

Yaniqui held back a snort. What a bland name. Must be a commercial deliveries ship. She felt the others gather behind her.

"This is a private ship, *529*. We have no wish to trade goods at this time."

"Be that as it may, we are looking to resecure company property that has recently been stolen. Property we have reason to believe is now located on your craft."

Hloban gave a short bark of a laugh. "We haven't stolen anything." He nearly smiled, more relaxed.

"Let me clarify—" Captain Jung was now more relaxed as well or at least having a good time. "This is *Transverser A00529* of the Akar Enterprises fleet. We're looking for a Wea Saavian, and have a permit to board any craft we have reason to believe she's on. Let's start gently now by turning on your camera."

# Chapter 29
## Hloban
## In Transit

Hloban looked at the others. Eeriva, still in a sleep shirt, swiftly pulled Yaniqui out of the frame. Hloban smoothed the worries out of his face and became a different, more confident person like magic. He switched on the camera.

"You're a long way from Akar Evion, aren't you?"

The screen flashed to life and an old man faced them. He wore the cream-and-white uniform Hloban had seen all over Akar Evion, but if there was any doubt, a watermark appeared in the bottom of the screen. Over the shoulder of Captain Jung loomed a large woman with a thick neck. She was not someone you would approach with a complaint—whether it was that she'd cooked your meal incorrectly or that the man she offed was your brother. Beyond them, there were bodies moving about the space, easily bigger than the entire *Caneille*. How many people, Hloban couldn't be sure. But it took only one to launch a heat-seeking missile.

"The business of Akar Enterprises is not limited to a single planet or star system. Our business takes us where it will. Now, itemize the beings on board with you."

Hloban looked over his shoulder at the others, then back into Jung's eyes. "Listen, I'd like to help you recover your lost property, but it stands that I'm a card-carrying member of the People's Liberation movement." Hloban felt Waquas stiffen beside him and glanced out of the corner of his eye. "So actually, I wouldn't like to help you. We didn't steal anyone, but that still doesn't mean if I had the last barrel of water in this godforsaken quadrant, we'd share it with your crew."

Hloban let himself get into the role he was playing and leaned toward the screen. "My uncle worked on Akar Evion for eight years. All we got back was a box of ashes." His voice pitched and ended. Their turn.

Jung looked like he'd expected a simple yes or no. "My condolences regarding your family member, sir. I can assure you though, those stories are often not what they seem. Doubtless, your uncle died of natural circumstances and Akar Enterprises did your family the courtesy of returning the remains." He cleared his throat sharply. "Now, Decree 7986QR from the Joint Council gives me full rights to ask: Who is on board?"

Hloban gave no names. "Myself, my cousin and his son, and two friends, all here on screen."

Jung nodded at someone to his side and looked forward intently.

"And the sixth body?"

Hloban fought to remain neutral.

With the swipe of the opposing captain's hand, he sent a video file over to the *Caneille*. Waquas cued it to play and there, on the screen, was the deadly dragon in midflight, dwarfing the fighter crafts around it. One pilot tried to maneuver under it and the dragon reached its long neck out to bite a wing. Upon impact, a quiver of force propelled through the air, lighting up the *Caneille* ever so briefly before the ship went invisible again.

"I don't know what that video's supposed to be of."

Jung smiled. "Even at this distance, we can run a heat analysis. There's a sixth body on board."

"My wife," Hloban said. If Adam snickered, Hloban was going to blast him out the hatch. "She's very ill and in bed."

"Very good, sir." The man nodded again at an aid. "We'll confirm such ourselves. Prepare to be boarded."

Eeriva and Waquas took positions immediately.

"I can't let you do that. I'm afraid it's contagious."

"As I said, earlier, we have a permit from the Joint Council to board any ship that has stolen property of Akar Enterprises. One of the benefits of paying taxes at the level we do on our lawful commercial endeavors. We will be mindful of our health."

Hloban never got to respond. Eeriva threw a switch and the screen went black. The *Caneille* lurched and he was blasted back. He was the only one that fell from the force. Apparently while he'd been dallying around pretending to be a badass, the others had been preparing. Keyad and Adam were strapped in, and Eeriva and Waquas were seated at the console. Waquas was rapidly plotting navigation while Eeriva kept tabs on the ship.

"What are you doing?" Hloban yelled from the ground, still caught off-balance.

Eeriva's answer came haltingly as she tried to focus on the task at hand. "This is a private ship. No defenses. No outer guns. They will board us if they get the opportunity. Our only option is to get away fast."

Waquas was already shaking his head. "We've been flying nonstop for days. The *Caneille* wasn't designed for a space race, and it's definitely not up for it now."

The craft agreed with a terrible groaning of metal as Waquas prepared to relaunch into Lightspeed+.

"What?" Adam shrieked. "We don't even have a single exterior gun?"

Yaniqui staggered out of the dormitory and lurched into Keyad. "Is the camera off? Can I come out now?"

Adam's snide answer was lost on Hloban. He knew what he had to do.

"Cut the speed by half. Hold the ship steady. Don't try to shake them. They'll attempt to communicate again if we put up a halfhearted flight. Line ourselves up with them when I say."

"So they can shoot us?" Eeriva spat.

"If we run, they'll shoot us for sure."

Then, Hloban was gone, into the back hall. He opened one of the floorboards and lifted up the small metal box he brought from Onlo. Yaniqui appeared.

"What's that, Hloban?"

He didn't reply but suited up. He didn't bother with the insulated lining or filling his air tank. He secured his gloves, his heavy breath already fogging up the tempered glass of his visor.

"Tell Eeriva to line us up now. Let them get close."

"What are you going to do?"

"Do it now!" The urgency in his voice scared Yaniqui and she bolted to the front room.

The *Caneille* felt like it was coasting on ice and slowed. Hloban hit the first air lock door and closed it behind him. He tethered himself to the iron ring and opened the door to space. Gravity evaporated under him and everything lifted. His magnetic boots buckled him fast to the floor and he aimed the Wipeout Con. It opened automatically with a flourish and reconfigured into a crossbow with one arrow. He felt it target and pull his arm sixteen degrees to the left at the Akarian ship. He took a breath, felt the span of two heartbeats, and pulled the trigger.

The arrow shot out of the tiny device, speeding toward the other ship. Hloban couldn't see anything, didn't even have to hope his aim was true. It hadn't yet landed, but his stomach fell. Of course, the Con would hit. It was designed to. Hloban closed the door around him and felt the pressure restabilize. His body had held itself together long enough. He shook with cold and adrenaline.

Out the back porthole, he watched *Transverser A00529*. It was as if someone smashed it with an enormous bat below the front viewpoint. The ship immediately flipped over itself. The dart was sure to pierce the hull. It could cut through titanium steel if needed and the moment the tiny capsule within the arrow burst, a chemical reaction would make the oxygen in the room all but vanish.

Hloban opened the helmet visor. Yaniqui looked at him in disbelief, her mouth hanging open. She followed him back to the living quarters. Hloban felt weightless, as if gravity hadn't yet secured its hold on him.

Everyone staring at the screen pivoted to stare at Hloban. "Shit," Eeriva said. "You're a murderer."

# Chapter 30

Adam
In Transit

Adam watched the *Transverser A00529* flip ass over front as if it were a racing car on Earth that blew a tire at deadly speed. His insides tightened instinctively at the sight. His brain was milliseconds behind as he realized what that kind of crash would do to a humanoid body. Or an animoid body. Or inanimate objects.

Waquas piloted the *Caneille* a safe distance away—most importantly out of the track the Akar ship was set to skid on through space for all eternity.

Hloban had pulled the trigger of something. One shot and he ended lives. One shot and it was over.

How fucking cool was that?

"What the fuck was that?" Eeriva bellowed.

"Just defending my craft." Hloban smoothed back a mess of unruly hair. He looked calm, a little nauseous, but all in all good for a civilian who had killed a ship full of Akar employees.

"You know what I mean. What was that weapon?"

Waquas's voice broke through the noise. "Did you have a

Wipeout Con on board this whole time?"

Eeriva looked like her eyes were going to bug out. "What if it had accidently been set off in here?"

"That was so fucking cool," Adam said. "Like a real space battle."

"Really, Adam? That's your takeaway from this?" Keyad looked disapprovingly at his son.

"I've only had it since Onlo," Hloban explained to Eeriva.

"You said you just got the cloak for the ship."

Hloban settled uncomfortably in a chair. It didn't seem to occur to him to take his suit off. "Well, I got both. Just in case." He looked up, resolve back. "And if you didn't notice, it was a good thing I did. Otherwise, we'd be boarded right now, they'd recapture Yaniqui, and the rest of us would be arrested for theft. Except Waquas."

Adam asked, "Why not Waquas?" but what he thought of as the adults ignored him. They bickered and Adam made eye contact with Yaniqui. Like everyone else, she looked a bit green around the gills.

"How do you think they found us?" Keyad asked.

Adam shook his head. "There wouldn't have been any chance to place a tracker on the ship—"

"It's a craft," Yaniqui corrected.

"—they didn't even know we were on Akar Evion until minutes before we left. Maybe our transmissions? Maybe they hacked our search history."

Keyad caught up to what they were saying. "Adam, that'd be impossible. That'd mean Akar had the ability to siphon the usage histories of every Wave user."

"We've got to leave these quadrants," Waquas said. "Hloban, are we still making for Earth?"

Eeriva threw her hands in disbelief and outrage. "Where the hell else could we go?"

But Hloban was at the console, no longer listening. He slid open a metal cabinet, pulled out a handful of cords, selected two, and wrenched them with a crunch.

"Dude, you could have just turned off the Wave."

Adam couldn't fall back asleep. He didn't know what the point was anyway. Who cared if he missed out on two hours and forty-five minutes of sleep?

Eeriva actually. Though she wasn't going back to bed anytime soon.

It was easier to go to the dormitory than listen to her berate Hloban. Waquas and Keyad were working to plot a less-direct route to Earth.

At the moment, Earth had as much appeal as a smushed banana. Adam wanted to stay in space. The adventure was fun. But there'd been no opportunities to network, job hunt, or blast off into his real life. It was finally hitting him that once he was home, he was back to square one.

Well, not totally, he'd now join the 0.0002 percent of Earth's population that had been to space. That had to count for something on job applications.

A secret journey to save the galaxy's most wanted person.

Adam set bolt upright, his blanket falling to his waist.

Would he ever even be able to tell anyone?

Oh gods, what if he'd never be able to tell anyone?

The door opened and a stripe of light fell across him. He put his arm up to block the bright lights.

The door shut.

"Ugh, are you masturbating again?"

"Jesus Christ, Yaniqui, that was one time. In the bathroom. And you didn't knock."

Adam punched his pillow and laid down. He heard Yaniqui undress in the dark and arrange herself in the bunk opposite his.

"Adam?"

"I am not touching myself. Get ahold of *your*self."

"I kind of can't believe Hloban killed those people."

Adam took a deep breath. "I know. Me too."

"Do you think it was the right thing to do?"

The pillow rustled in his ear as Adam turned his head. He tried to make out anything about Yaniqui in the dark but couldn't see her shape, much less her expression.

"Well, those guys were going to board us and enslave you again, right?"

"I guess so."

It went quiet for so long Adam thought Yaniqui had drifted off.

"It still feels like a waste. They were doing bad things, but they still died because of me. A lot of people have gotten hurt since the start of this."

Adam couldn't see her, but he could read the sadness in her voice. "I know, Yani." He looked up at the ceiling. "I'm sorry about your mom. And I'm sure there are others you're thinking about." He swallowed, looking for the right words. "But it's not your responsibility to keep others safe. You didn't set this sequence of events into action."

She gave a humorless chuckle. "Well, I kind of did."

Adam made a curious noise in his throat.

"I was the one who got me and Maemi discovered." She told him briefly about Sario, about working in the infirmary on 4,278, and about the appearance of the bounty hunter. "And I *have* made decisions all along the way—if I'd cooperate, if I'd try to escape, who I asked for help. Boarding this craft even."

Adam shook his head, then realized she couldn't see him either. "How can you be held accountable for choosing between two bad options if you're in an impossible situation?"

He heard a smile in her voice. "You know, Adam, you're all right."

He smiled in response.

"But try not to jack yourself off while I'm in here."

"Fuck you," he muttered, rolled over, and went to sleep.

The Wave was gone so they couldn't do video calls with their family, but they could still receive essential messages on the *Caneille*'s backup communicator. It was ancient so Hloban wasn't worried about it being tracked. Waquas called Adam over to hear the latest transmission.

"This is Jerimiah Thompson from Immigration Services. I'm trying to get in touch with Adam Jayul. His leave from Earth for a, uh, vacation/rescue expired five business days ago and we have no records of his return to Earth—"

Adam looked up sharply at his dad who appeared at the mention of his son's name.

The voice, scratchy through the expanses of space, said, "We'll need a formal notification of whereabouts and reason for delay. If this order is not followed, Adam Jayul will be subject to a fine of up to $31,500."

Keyad sent a voice message to Amanda asking her if she could collect and fill out the paperwork. He sent along their current coordinates. They were a week out from the Jupiter Station. An hour later they got a message back from Loera. Amanda had called Loera's assistant, Mari, for help drafting some of the language, but Loera insisted she take it on herself. Loera said in her message it would be beneficial to indicate without a doubt that Adam intended to return and would he like her to secure an interview at one of her friends' companies?

Adam indicated that he did indeed appreciate the offer. Eight hours later, he was invited to submit an application with Green Timber Fabrication.

"What the fuck?" Adam stated baldly. "I thought Loera meant an interview with one of her cool friends—not a manufacturing company."

Eeriva tilted her head and looked at Adam out of the side of her eye. "You should be grateful."

"I mean, come on, is this what Loera thinks of me?"

Eeriva shrugged. "If I had a company, I'd hire you."

"Wow, Eeriva, that's actually kind. Thank you."

"Wouldn't put you in charge of trash collection though."

"And there it is."

Adam sat to record his cover letter. He got as far as recounting his various internships when things went wrong.

"—and as part of the team for the summer, I programmed—"

"*All* I'm saying is you have to tell her I'm an adult before we get there."

Adam tried speaking louder. "—ensuring a more streamlined system—"

"She'll get to know you when we get to Earth."

"I don't want to get to know *your wife*—I'm supposed to be your wife, remember? If you would have a little dignity and stop pretending to her that I'm some innocent kid that's never had a wet dream about you—"

Adam swung around in a rage. "Do you two *mind?* I'm *trying* to send an interview piece to this shit company so Earth knows I want to go back to their shit planet. And Yaniqui, no one wants to hear about your sex dreams. So, if you don't mind—" Adam turned back to the console to see that the recording timed out and automatically sent.

"Goddamn holy shit!"

# Chapter 31

D-68
The Catchment, Earth

D-68 takes extra care with the tiny body. A flop of brown hair falls across the small creature's smooth forehead. This one was not taken in with promises of substances. While the others have the look of a peaceful, drug-induced sleep, the child is clammy and troubled.

'vo sees D-68 holding the child. "I had to hit that one on the head. Get him strapped in with the rest. It doesn't matter if he wakes a little early."

"Take him?"

"I didn't mean to, big guy. He must have followed his dad or his big brother out."

D-68 has never been so close to a humanoid kit, and especially not an Earthling kit.

"Come on, let's finish up, I'm supposed to go see Leggs pronto."

Did he have the words needed to ask his question? To argue that perhaps the kits at least should be left out of it?

'vo sees his hesitation. "I know, it's…not right, but the kid saw everything. He can't stay here."

D-68 continues to stand, holding the kid.

"Aww, come on. Earthlings act like this is such a special place while all the rest of us have been moved around. That's part of the galaxy ecosystem. And not just the money we're making—where would any of our peoples be if we didn't randomly move around to evolve and intermix? This boy could go out there and have a better life. He could stay here and die tomorrow. It's all random chance."

D-68 takes a step toward the spacecraft.

"Okay," 'vo says. "I wasted enough time talking philosophy with you. Leggs is going to be pissed. You finish up."

D-68 continues toward the craft but never within sight of the windows, where the Earthling pilot can see. He hears 'vo recede into the woods. Looking around carefully, he takes the kit and hides him behind a bush. He cares not for Earthlings but moving a kit is taboo. As if doing so means someone would come and take his own kits from their home.

The Earthling grumbles about the time and they get the rest of the humanoids strapped in. D-68 watches the man place gray plastic coverings over the humanoids' hands. It shrinks on contact, holding them bound. D-68 gets off the craft and heads into the trees opposite where he stashed the human. Once the ship is out of sight, he retrieves the kit.

He feels small and vulnerable in his arms. D-68 wonders at the life of this child, at his future. Yes, it would have been wrong to move him from his people, even if it was a family member who now speeds away, likely to never return. He walks along the fence away from where he and 'vo usually come and go, and lays the child on gravel. Spindly plants push through in some places. The child looks cold and D-68 frets. He gathers dried leaves from the forest and surrounds the boy, like he would put moss around a kit.

He starts back. Dawn will arrive soon. He smells the coming scent of 'vo—a little spicy, a little exhausted. 'vo emerges through the fence.

"You're up next."

When D-68 doesn't move, he speaks again, "Leggs wants you. Go now, D."

D-68 moves slowly through the Catchment pathways. He wishes

he could leap and climb along the structures, but they are too frail to support him. He follows the ghost of 'vo's scent to the dwelling of the many-legged one. The boy translator is already there, must always be there. He is bigger than the boy D-68 hid, and solemn. The creature *tsks*.

"Take this," the boy says, "to the southern regulators tower."

D-68 reaches for the small metal box. It burns across his nose. Their technology always does.

The many-legged one quivers. "Attach it to the underside of the guardhouse. Make sure no one sees you. When you're done, leave that place. If you do well, tomorrow night I will have food for you."

It takes a long time to reach the tower. The black of night has a smooth quality to it now. Light will soon mingle and banish the black. It is a relief when D-68 arrives. He climbs effortlessly and sticks the little box just below the room on top. He hears voices above and wonders if the box is a recording device. D-68 is rarely impressed, but when he saw a holo for the first time, playing out the movements and sound that had already finished happening in life, it left a mark on him.

D-68 climbs down and goes to the forest. He will visit the stream and fill his belly before he sleeps.

Thunder rolls across the sky. It is unlike the boom of the Earth rains. It is loud and deadly. D-68 looks behind, terrified. Through the trees, he sees smoke pour out of the regulators tower. Flames lick the windows. The entire top shakes and breaks apart, cracked open like a lizard's egg. One of the sides falls away, the sound of concrete cracking is clear and clean to D-68's ear, but it is all unnatural.

The box. The box. D-68 knows it has to be the box he left.

There are screams. From the tower or below, D-68 does not know. D-68 does not eat meat. He does not kill if it can be helped. Wiping out lives without knowing what his actions did is a shock to him.

He drops to his knees and shakes and whimpers and thinks of his own life, gone. He wants to go home. Recently he has grown numb to the shocking nature of his experiences. In this moment, he is deeply vulnerable once again.

A crack in the darkness makes D-68 jump to his feet and take a defensive stance.

# Chapter 32

Lozen
The Catchment, Earth

In the ever-so-slowly lightening dark of night was a huge shadow that defied expectation. The videos of slaughter, the GIA's narrative of violence—all of it whispered in Lozen's ear to shrink and cower. If he should touch her, even without malicious intent, she could be squashed to a pulp. It took everything within Lozen not to run. No dream of the big city tickled her mind, no sense of justice kept her rooted to her spot; rather only the internal instinct of all small animals to go silent and still, and hope the predator passes by. Lozen was saved from decision by a huge flash and a bang that rang through the sky. She took her eyes off D-68, the new development more terrifying than the last.

*Oh, fuck, it's the whole tower.* Lozen's mouth dropped open and adrenaline—already high—made her stagger forward like a silly girl, arm outstretched, as if she could catch the tower before it fell. The flaming regulators tower, already buckling, sent a snarl of steel through the night air. Shouts of surprise came from the houses below. It fell sluggishly and landed with a terrible crash that made Lozen jump back.

Another bombing. As terrible as it was, Lozen could finally let out a breath. It happened again, and not to her.

The form in the darkness moved by her side and Lozen spun to find D-68 watching her. The hard casing of his skin—his scales, no, an insect-like shell—covered most of his body. Though bug came to mind, he had no antenna, no strange protrusions. He didn't remind her of Leggs or any other animoids in the Catchment. He was in a class of his own.

He grabbed for her.

Lozen willed her body to move and flinched right. It was enough. She got her legs under her and ran blindly into the woods. The heat of the bombing faded quickly, but so did the yells for water and the screams of people. He wasn't attuned to moving through the trees like she was. Lozen could easily hear D-68's clumsy movements behind her. Steps away? Was she putting any distance between them? She couldn't turn and look, couldn't risk giving up any ground. She stumbled over brush but used a tree to catch herself and launch in another direction.

D-68 collided with the same tree she had pushed off. A splinter cracked the air and the tree toppled, giving up its life with a groan and crash. A whine escaped Lozen as her feet gave out from under her. She tripped fast, falling on her hands, and a pain in her right knee made her cry out. The enormous sound of cracking wood still rang in her ears, forcing her to roll hard to the side. She felt her bag catch on something. She had forgotten she even had it on and fought desperately to slip it from her shoulder, free herself, and run. Lozen got as far as her knees and crawled, painfully slow.

The nutty scent of acorns filled the small clearing. Still on the ground, Lozen rolled to her back, scrambling a few feet farther for good measure. Her tense, painful chest fought to remind her to breathe. She couldn't help but look at the coming reason for her demise—to see how much longer she had to live.

D-68 scooped a handful of acorns up and tossed them in his mouth. Lozen couldn't see them in his large clawed hands because he scraped them off the ground with the under mulch of the forest—leaves, bracken, and flecks of mud. Heedless of any of it, D-68 knocked another handful back. He looked like a starving man eating the meal he had been longing for in the heartbeats between hunger pains.

A man? What made her think that? He was nothing like a man. He was a monster.

Lozen had gotten up early to retrieve a cache of acorns from the woods that she had gathered and hidden the previous fall. She tried to sort the rotten ones out in the dark, gave up, and put everything in her bag to trade at the market when the sun was up. Her mind couldn't help but consider what would have happened had she not had them with her. Then again, she wouldn't have been up and out so early in the morning.

D-68 ate with abandon. Lozen wondered if he had forgotten she was there when he cast an eye in her direction. She knew instantly that he would have given anything not to have let her see him like that, but he was too overcome with hunger. The sudden vulnerability tinged with a need to deflect and control the situation made Lozen speak.

"Did you bomb that tower?"

She thought he understood her, but he focused on picking up the last few of the tree nuts and crushed them between his broad teeth. Then, he stood.

That forced Lozen to stagger to her own feet. Even fully erect, she gaped up at him like a child. A wild thought flicked across her mind. *What did humanoids look like to him? Like soft, strange amphibians?* But she didn't have time for such musings. The feeling of his angry eyes upon her was too much. She spun and broke into a run.

Though the forest was the home of her ancestors, and D-68 was molded for another world entirely, he maneuvered in front of her easily and cut her off. She pivoted and balked when he got in front of her again. His stiff and ungainly gait made it all the more infuriating that he could be faster than she was.

"You're a monster," she said, hoping the venom in her voice gave him pause. "You killed those people."

"You. Monster, you all," he said. "Weak one accuse me. Your people."

"How can you say that? You came to our planet to terrorize it."

"Brought I here."

"Yes," her voice was near hysterical. "You were brought here because you killed a human. You can't kill me too. The GIA knows I'm out here."

D-68 bellowed, his rage emulating in snarls. Lozen's eyes widened and a hand rocketed to her mouth. She bent over just in time for foul-smelling sick to come up her throat. She couldn't help but expose her neck as she heaved, even though an enemy stood nearby. The thought sent shivers down her back as she convulsed.

It took a while before she was able to come out of her crouch and wipe her mouth with the back of her hand. D-68 moved upwind of her. His nose couldn't wrinkle in disgust, but she could almost read his mind—the smell of humans is frightful.

"GIA know what?" he demanded.

"They know you're somewhere around the Catchment and that you keep terrorizing us. First the handout station—that was where we got food, by the way," she said, still fearful but with heat coming back to her voice. A wave of smoke came on the wind and obscured the scent of her vomit.

D-68 looked genuinely taken aback at what Lozen said. "No. No me." He gave a strange shake of his head.

"They're going to catch you. I saw you running from the guard tower just as it exploded. You killed those people."

D-68 rushed at her. Lozen crouched down, fearing the worst, but he stopped, like a bear staking claim in its territory but not going in for the actual fight.

"No me," he said again.

"What do you even want? Are you killing people because you hate us? Do you want the GIA to bring you back to your planet?"

He let out a low, involuntarily moan and lumbered his head side to side.

She sniffed the wetness in her nose disgustingly. "So, that's what you want? You want to go home?"

"Not know. Not kill." He paused and considered. What he said next took great effort to speak aloud. "Many-legged one."

Lozen stepped back, startled. "Leggs? He's behind the

bombings?" Lozen shook her head slowly. That didn't surprise her, but it scared her. "Why would he do that?"

"Hate." It is one word, but D-68 said it bitterly.

They stood quietly for a moment. Lozen could walk away, be done with all of this. Tell the Karmas and the GIA that she was giving up. But she was so close to the truth. To actually being able to help her neighbors in the Catchment.

"Follow." D-68 turned his back on Lozen. She licked her bottom lip, considering her options. Trusting him seemed like the worst idea on the planet, and yet, Lozen couldn't do anything else. Not if she really wanted to know.

She broke into a soft jog to catch up. It was a funny feeling, walking through the woods alongside D-68. She didn't bother trying to make small talk. She could barely understand him about the important stuff. And what would she ask anyway? If he knew any recipes for acorns?

Eventually, he crouched. Lozen instantly did the same and glanced around to see who they were hiding from. There, the clearing. Not the one where she met Agent Tril, but a clearing where she and Monte once pretended to train martial arts in. They'd seen an old movie and it was all they could talk about that summer.

In the middle was a ship. Lozen covered her open mouth with her hand and peered urgently through the bush.

Two animoids rolled barrels into a nondescript ship. And there, waving them in, was Agent Velazquez.

# Chapter 33
## Ippa
## Jupiter Station

Nothing changed for Ippa immediately except her perception of herself. She slept in the same bunk and ate the same food the station offered her. Her parents didn't know about her massive downfall, and neither did Bel, Professor Jinu, or anyone else. That Ippa was no longer a student, and about to become a migrant worker on a Podunk planet was surreal. She could almost forget it.

Until the forms came.

*What was the trade of choice on your home planet?*

*Technological Assemblages.*

*Do you have experience growing plants?*

*No.*

*Can your species tolerate exposure to high levels of lead? Radiation?*

*Incompatible with the two listed.*

Mrs. Potscha spent an extensive session with Ippa asking questions about what type of technology her planet created and whether Ippa herself had experience building weapons or defense mechanisms. Ippa revealed that items were not designed on her planet, only manufactured. Her parents and extended family mainly assembled oxygenators and other items related to spacecraft life support. Ippa tried to summon a respectable level of pride for her parents' professions in manufacturing, but it was clear Mrs. Potscha was disappointed.

"I was thinking though, my labor contribution could be to write an ethnography."

Mrs. Potscha shook her head with a scrunch in the middle of her face, curls waving. She didn't even respond, the idea was so worthless.

"I could track things from the refugees' point of view." The enthusiasm in Ippa's voice was real. "I could collect stories from their past and record their responses to Earth life and culture."

"We already know what they think of Earth," Mrs. Potscha said, exasperated.

Ippa resigned herself to the knowledge that any academic work would be on her own. She would do whatever manual labor was expected of her to relieve her debt. She cried quietly in her bunk and held tightly to the thought of the scientists, explorers, and anthropologists that faced hardship. After all, Demoran Nix himself was stranded on a rural planet for a quarter of his life. When he finally made it off the planet on a grain barge, he brought the leaf scrolls with his foundational work recorded on them. This was not the end of Ippa's story. She was going to manifest the crisps out of her future and do exactly what she'd always planned on doing with her life—find excellence in research and understand the universe!

Still, Ippa was unenthusiastic about her current choices and casually added one more option to her list—go above Mrs. Potscha's head.

Two Earth ambassadors were currently lodging at the Jupiter Station after long assignments elsewhere. Ippa saw them at meal times, but she sensed a resentment, a coldness of some sort from both the women. She figured it was an exhaustion of languages, accents, and other cultures. They were on their way home, what did they need to talk with more aliens for?

Despite this, Ippa thought it prudent to seek them out and try to build a stronger connection. It could make all the difference.

There were only three day/night cycles left before the journey to Earth when Ippa saw one Earth ambassador by chance, walking down the central functioning hallway.

"Excuse me. Pardon me."

Was it Ippa or was the woman pretending not to hear?

"I wanted a moment with you. I was recently a student at The Shou and I'm traveling to Earth for a research project."

The ambassador looked tentatively over her shoulder and smiled. "Enjoy the journey to Earth."

"Actually…"

The ambassador's eyes narrowed.

"I was hoping I could talk to you more about Earth. See, I am trying to compile some information from an academic point of view. I have already talked with many of the refugees and have important case interviews set up on Earth. One is with a family that is going to be taking in an endangered species to live with them." Ippa didn't mention that was the only thing she had set up.

The woman's face softened instantly. "So, you hope to meet with these individuals and gather information? It sounds like you have access to an especially unique case."

Ippa was relieved the ambassador understood. "That's right. I hope to submit it to Shou University, where I studied, and bolster their information on Earth for other scholars to utilize. Firsthand interviews are lacking in their library."

"And the rare species? Is it the Wea Saavian?" the ambassador ventured.

"Well, I'm not sure," Ippa said. She saw a news story about a Wea Saavian's discovery, but the poor woman was owned by Akar.

"Just between us, the Wea Saavian escaped. All of Earth's diplomats receive notice when special cases like hers are taken on."

Ippa lit up. A Wea Saavian. That would be pure research gold. "It could be her," she said, hopefully. Anything to move this along.

The ambassador mulled, finger on her chin. "This could certainly be useful research that could help us build relationships with other planets. We know little of how Earth culture is perceived by others," she said.

Ippa felt relieved for the first time since she had left the university. Earth was like anywhere else—it was who you knew.

"The other ambassador and I are leaving on our private ship at 0630. Could you be ready to go with us?"

"Yes, of course." Ippa struggled to keep her voice down. "How long is the journey to Earth?"

"It's about two Earth weeks. No interstellar highway out here, I'm afraid. Get your bags packed. It would be helpful if you could purchase some supplies from the canteen. It's a small craft and we weren't counting on a third passenger." She smiled apologetically.

"Of course." Ippa quickly calculated what the last of her funds would get her.

"It would also behoove you not to mention this to anyone else. We don't want any issues to halt our departure."

"You mean others in the labor program might be jealous?"

The ambassador hesitated for a brief second. "Yes, that's right. Others will be upset at this special treatment we're giving you, but you have so much to offer in return."

Finally, someone who understood. Ippa went back to her bunk entirely relieved and spent her last few waking hours on the Jupiter Station recording her good fortune and drafting interview questions on her handheld.

In the middle of the sleep shift, Ippa rolled quietly out of the bed, mindful not to wake Kim or the others. She slept dressed in her tunic so all she had to do was tie her boots on. Her bags were already packed. She paused at the door wondering what the women would think when they found her gone.

Ippa continued down the corridors toward the docking area. In retrospect, she wished she had taken more advantage of her time at the Jupiter Station. She was such an emotional wreck, she hadn't done any formal interviews with the staff. Ippa resolved that when she left the Sol System—which she would do in a blaze of field study glory—she would arrange for a bit of extra time at the Station to do things properly. It would be a good bookend to her experience, and perhaps even worth a book itself.

In the spacecraft bay, the two ambassadors readied a small vessel. It was by far the tiniest spacecraft Ippa had ever boarded. The woman she had spoken to was the taller and older of the two. Ippa was impressed two relatively young women had secured such prestigious positions as intersteller ambassadors. They nodded curtly at her and indicated she load her bags and strap in. Ippa felt the thrill of departure. She would have liked to wave out the window to someone. In fact, where were the safety checkers? So far, the station had been meticulous to the last detail.

The engine purred to life and she heard the safety locks unclick. The craft jarred as it rolled to the transition point and then disembarked into the absolute nothingness of space. It made sense to Ippa that ambassadors would also be technologically savvy beings. What if they had to address problems while out visiting other planets or make an escape after difficult negotiations went awry? Ippa's head buzzed with theories. She had not felt this inspired in a long time. She wished her handheld was handy, but she had stowed her personal bags and food supplies.

The two at the console conferred, but Ippa couldn't hear them from where she was strapped in, then the younger ambassador came back by Ippa and grabbed her by the arm.

Ippa tried to pull away. "Excuse me," she said.

The ambassador didn't let go. It was as if Ippa's mind blipped out, but she was still staring at the woman. Disbelief. *No, I'm fine,* she reassured herself.

Ippa struggled when the woman didn't release her. "Stop it. Let go of me." Ippa looked for the other woman, but she was piloting the craft. "She said I was allowed."

"They said you were allowed," the woman corrected. "But when you curse me tonight, you can use she/her. Let's get you down below."

Despite her slight stature, the woman was much stronger than Ippa. She unbuckled Ippa from her seat. They wrestled back and forth. Ippa's head slammed against a wall. Her ears went hollow and she saw dots before her eyes. Move, move, move anywhere. She felt along the wall, looking for something to hold on to and fight back with.

The woman used Ippa's disorientation to unroll a square of

standard gray carpet. Underneath was a round metal door. She opened it, hauled Ippa over, and rolled her in.

Ippa free-fell for the briefest of moments, but it was long enough to know her entire life was over. She had made a miscalculation. Perhaps a few of them.

The woman jumped down after her.

*Why don't I know her name?* Ippa wondered. She struggled to back away from the stranger.

The woman pulled on Ippa's shoulders to raise her.

Ippa slashed at her face with her nails.

The woman deflected her easily and punched Ippa in the stomach.

"No, you can't do this," Ippa slurred.

"There's no need for all that." The woman grabbed Ippa's ankle and harshly clipped a heavy shackle to her. She slithered out of reach and made her way up a ladder, back to the surface.

Ippa was furious at being overtaken so easily. Her actions were slow. She posed no threat. Anyone else would have sensed the coming danger, but Ippa was so blinded by her pride and self-confidence that she didn't understand she had slid further and further into vulnerability.

# Chapter 34
## Hloban
## Sol System

Jupiter was all but a dot in the sky. The station itself was long lost beside the behemoth gas giant, and Hloban wondered when he'd have opportunity to leave the solar system again. Every time, he wondered if it was the last time. Not that he worried about dying a premature death, he thought fate had something else in mind, but all ties to life outside Earth would be lost to him. Then, he would simply become a man who lived somewhere he didn't belong.

Standing at the console, eyes on the rear cam, he shifted to accommodate Eeriva who sat and began typing with a businesslike manner. He peeked over her shoulder and saw she was sending reports to Earth. She was a good executive officer.

Fortunately, captains were allowed to be a bit more eccentric. He sighed. Maybe he'd go work out some more. Increase the settings to prepare for full Earth gravity. He made for the hall to get his exercise clothes from his cubby, when he saw Adam and Yaniqui sitting next to each other at the bolted-down table. Hloban was surprised because he hadn't heard them talking.

He pretended to check the fastenings on a vent and peered over at them again. He spied a small metallic sheen in Yaniqui's left ear and Adam's right ear. They were listening to something together. Yaniqui had tied her black curls back, eyes on the book in front of her. Adam scrolled through his device.

There. Adam clicked a new song and his eyes flicked to Yaniqui to see her response. She looked back at Adam and gave a half shrug and nod in acceptance. Jealously bloomed in Hloban's chest. The screw from the vent came apart in his hand as he realized he had been loosening rather than fastening it as he watched Adam and Yaniqui. He retrieved the electric screwdriver from an under-floor compartment and refitted the piece of metal, securing the vent. He checked on the others again. Yaniqui pointed to something in her book and watched Adam's face as he read over her shoulder.

Despite his wife, despite what he'd tried to make Yaniqui believe, he wanted to tear the book away and toss it to the floor. No, not even that. He wanted to be in a dark room, free of responsibilities, free from all thoughts of the future, and just have Yaniqui's length pressed against his.

"Getting hard there, huh?"

Hloban startled and pulled back the drill. "I beg your pardon?" He turned round on Eeriva.

"You can't fasten that screw so tightly or it's bound to strip the inside."

Hloban gave a jerk of a nod and packed up the equipment. He refused to look in the table's direction before departing to his locker.

He couldn't be mad. He had told Yaniqui he was unavailable. And he rightly was.

They'd all been living in close quarters. He'd seen it before. People could grow to hate each other, but constant exposure could also bring people together quickly. Was that what was happening to Adam and Yani?

He undid the fasteners on his locker—no one was concerned enough to set a lock on this odyssey. Once you snuck into Akar Evion and watched their minions perish in space, there was no point in protecting socks from your crewmates. Hloban changed quickly, ducked into the exercise room, and shut the door. It was miniscule, just big enough for someone like Waquas to have a few feet of clearance on either side of his outstretched hands. For Hloban, it was comfortable.

The lights cued down and up as a running path along the mountains of Kervestki appeared. The amber-yellow sky contrasted sharply with the jade-studded rocks. Hloban set to it and tried not to let his mind wander back to Yaniqui—it was both too painful and too enticing—but it was impossible. Everything was about her. For the millionth time, he wondered why he'd been split from her and his planet. Five Wea Saavians left. Six, if Nica was still alive.

He pushed into his run and tried to soften his mind, but all the thoughts of Wea Saa and what could have been kept flooding back. The last of the Wea Saavians, nearly all accounted for on this tiny ship.

There could be more. Obani may have kids. Yaniqui could have kids even. She could have kids with Adam. Flashes of sorrow and ingenuity seized his brain.

His head snapped up as he realized what had to be done.

What if Adam and Yaniqui were meant to be together? What if they fell in love? That'd justify finding Yaniqui and bringing her back to Earth. Loera would rest easier at night. Would he feel less guilty for breaking Yani's heart? Yes. What about his own? Never.

The machine automatically decreased from a sprint to a jog as the incline shifted upward. Purple clouds gathered as he climbed higher on the mountain. Hloban reached out, palm up and the speed increased to a sprint once more.

The question was, could Hloban live with Yaniqui moving on? It was what he had done, even though he'd never fully reconciled his loss. Never stopped mourning her. Hloban had made a choice to find family elsewhere, but that didn't mean she wasn't his. And therein lay a responsibility so deep it could cut—the happiness of someone else.

Hloban considered Adam objectively. He was smart, driven, a Wea Saavian who knew far too little of his people's traditions. Though they looked so similar—clearly of the same tribe—Adam and

Yani had grown up with vastly different beliefs. Yaniqui was set in the Wea Saavian way of long expectation and acceptance. Adam was an Earthling who believed you could bend destiny to your will.

Hloban slowed the machine and jogged, plodding ahead but going nowhere.

It was settled.

After his run, he'd towel off with the cleansing powder. He'd sip some water, stretch out, and prepare to do all he could to make Adam and Yaniqui fall in love.

*Fuck.*

# Chapter 35
Adam
Earth

Adam called Yaniqui over from her chore of wiping out each magnetic cabinet, something Eeriva assigned her. She walked over to join him at the screen and control panel. Adam pointed—hovering in the black of space was an ever-growing, bright marble.

"It's so blue," Yaniqui said astonished.

Hloban was clicking something on the console but turned and smiled. "I told you it was something. Who knew that could be way out here? Most of the water you see has salt in it. We can't drink it, but a lot of animals live in it. You can drive a boat for weeks without seeing land," Hloban said.

"Have you?"

"Hmm? No. We do not live near any of the oceans. We do live near the Great Lakes, which are big enough."

Adam's dad said, "Here, humanity grew up next to the waterways. The oceans were once full of food and they were integral to colonizing the entire planet. Complete planetary exploration and expansion gave Earthlings the momentum to get off planet, eventually leading to rediscovery."

Adam looked up sharply. "What do you mean rediscovered?"

Yaniqui broke in, "He said rediscovered because obviously somewhere along the way the humans on Earth forgot their technology, including how they got there in the first place."

Yaniqui still annoyed the crap out of him, but he didn't have time for that. "Wait, what? In the first place?"

"After humans landed on Earth, something happened," Keyad said. "Maybe their craft broke and they didn't have the technology to fix it. Whatever the case, over time the knowledge was forgotten and people could move only as fast as they could walk until they invented other means. Wind-powered ships were instrumental in raising the quality of life."

Adam spoke quickly, "You mean Earthlings didn't start there?"

Yaniqui broke in, as if she couldn't help herself. "There were only nine base planets with Intelligent life, the Original Nine. Everything spread from there. Wea Saa wasn't one of the Original Nine either, but it was populated early, then isolated for a long time."

"Oh really," Adam said, still skeptical. "When did humans land on Earth?"

"Approximately two hundred thousand Earth years ago," Waquas said.

Adam's eyebrows shot up and he looked out the window at his home.

"This is absurd," Adam said. "I went to college. I've read pretty much anything I could get my hands on about life off Earth. Why haven't I heard of this or the Original Nine?"

Waquas looked away from the blue planet. "Precisely because you're reading about life off Earth. No one off-planet would think to write down Earth's history. And belief in this history is hard for Earthlings. It's in the interest of governments and religions to go along with public assumption that Earthlings evolved on that planet."

"But that's propaganda," Adam said.

"Yes," said Waquas. "It is."

The transmitter beeped. "Hello, Loera speaking," rang crisply through the space.

Yaniqui went to the bath capsule. Adam wasn't surprised. She wasn't ready for any of this but especially not that. She asked him yesterday what Loera looked like. He had said Loera was older than Hloban, so she'd be quite a bit older than Yaniqui. Adam made a point to mention how hot Loera was. And that she was smart. And had lots of money. And that everybody liked her. She had to know how it was. Adam drifted into the dormitory. He could imagine the call now. *How are you doing, how is the ship, how is that dangerous sexy girl you picked up in the middle of the galaxy?*

"Winslow Space-Earth Station here. Ship name and register number please."

"Well met, Winslow Station. *Caneille ES12* here."

"Prepare to land at 0935 hours."

Everyone strapped in as the Earth spiraled closer and closer. The huge oceans receded in the distance and browns and greens burst into view. They steadily formed into a landscape, then individual trees and buildings. Lower in their descent, there were thousands of moving parts to see—vehicles, people, lights, low-flying ships.

Waquas landed at the direction of Winslow Space-Earth Station. A man on the ground waved them through to a giant spaceship hangar. Waquas guided them into place and the ship gave a final shudder. They off-loaded into a holding area with four Earthlings inside.

Two women held guns at the ready but with smiles on their faces. "Welcome to Earth. And welcome home."

"What are those hairy beasts?" Yaniqui blurted. She was looking down curiously.

Indeed, a man and a third woman held ropes attached to two short hairy beasts. One wagged a tail. The other licked the side of his mouth, exposing a row of pointed teeth. Yaniqui flinched.

"It's called a dog," Adam said. "They're friendly."

"But not while they're working. Excuse me," the man said.

One of the armed women walked to the wall and touched markers on a screen. She checked off each step of their arrival. *Docking* and *greeting* were marked off. *Ship search* was in progress. A little dog face appeared next to that one.

While they waited, Keyad and Hloban tried to answer Yaniqui's questions. Adam listened intently; he didn't realize he had the same ones.

"Every time an alien decides to settle on Earth, its status grows in the eyes of the Joint Council. When especially rare or vulnerable species choose Earth, Earth receives funds from IERR, but also builds their case to become a formal part of the Council instead of a nonparticipatory member," Hloban said.

"That didn't bother you when you moved here?" Yaniqui asked.

"No. I needed a home and I wanted to be with other Wea Saavians."

The speaker near the exit blared. "Adam, Keyad, are you there?"

"Mom," Adam said, shocked. "How are you even doing this?"

"Oh, thank goodness! I wanted to get to you right away. I called the operator and begged that they put me through. I've missed you so much."

Adam blushed. "We missed you too, Mom."

"Was going off-planet all you thought it would be? Was it an adventure? Do you feel like this will help you get a job?"

Adam heard a chuckle. The dog team was looking amused. Eeriva coughed, but for once in her life didn't say anything.

Keyad stepped in. "Amanda, we miss you too. Adam would love to answer all your questions when we're back. Winslow has us on a tight schedule."

"Oops! Goodbye!"

One of the attendants said, "Aww, you shouldn't have rushed her. Moms are a special thing."

Adam smiled despite his humiliation and looked over at Yaniqui to share the joke, but she was decidedly looking away.

After the rounds of paperwork, interviews, and a final medical clearance at Winslow, Adam and the group headed back to the *Caneille*. They were finished with the bureaucracy. It was time to go home. Once inside, Adam noticed for the first time how horrendous it smelled after housing six adults for months, recycling the same air.

Everyone was in good spirits and talking when Eeriva picked up her bag.

"I'll stay here at Winslow and get a ride on my own."

At that point in the trip, Adam had almost forgotten that Eeriva wasn't one of them. Keyad thanked Eeriva profusely and Eeriva wished him luck. She nodded at Adam and whispered to Yaniqui on her way out, "Don't let them push you around."

Then she was gone.

Waquas took them up into the air and the landscape turned green as they left the immediate capital. The short ride out lasted much longer than Adam expected, but he was used to zooming at Lightspeed+. Yaniqui positioned herself in front of the larger porthole, not asking questions but drinking it all in. Waquas landed the ship on a huge concrete foundation surrounded by wilderness, within view of only his small home. There was a flurry of activity as everyone congregated at the door, leaving all bags behind for now.

Despite his earlier embarrassment, Adam raced out and gave his mom a huge bear hug. "It was amazing. Thanks for letting me go." The fresh spring air felt alive. He took a deep breath, his arms still wrapped around his mom.

"You didn't need my permission, Adam. I just wanted to help you be sure. And look at all that you've done."

Adam looked back to introduce Yaniqui to his mom. He found Waquas checking over the ship and Hloban was tightly locked with Obani. But Yaniqui lingered inside.

She took a tentative step out into the warm sunlight. Her eyes flitted across the scene and took in the tall, budding trees, more trees than could be counted. It finally hit Adam what an oasis Earth was. The wind blew through the trees and Yaniqui shivered. His feet stuck a little because the ground was freshly damp from the rain. He had already been awake longer than his normal day and night cycle, but he felt another wave of energy as Yaniqui walked down the ramp. Everyone looked up at her.

"Yaniqui." Hloban touched her shoulder. "I'd like to introduce my wife, Loera." And there Loera was, in brightly colored glasses and a thin finely woven sweater, cut along the top to show smooth shoulders. He watched Yani look her over. Yes, she was older, and extremely fine wrinkles bordered her eyes, but in an instant anyone who met her knew she was one of those women with an unbreakable string that pulled her through life to become who she always knew she would be. She got stronger and more elegant with each new year and adventure.

Yaniqui turned hastily back to Hloban and blurted, "Can I get a dog?"

Loera stiffened. "Yaniqui, welcome to Earth. Well, I thought you were a little girl."

"Why did you think I was a little girl? The clothes didn't fit, you know."

Loera casually put her arm through Hloban's. "I guess because Hoban always talked about you as if you were a child."

"We were both children when we were first betrothed like ages ago. Anyway, that's not how you say his name."

Loera tilted her face toward Hloban, confusion evident.

"Yani, she has an Earth accent," Hloban said.

Adam had noticed the subtle difference in how Yaniqui addressed Hloban, but he pronounced it the same as Loera. He didn't know it was wrong.

"I thought maybe she'd like to know she wasn't saying your name right. So anyway, where can I get one of those animals?"

Loera dropped her voice needlessly—everyone was looking at the trio anyway. "Do I really say your name wrong?" she asked Hloban.

Hloban paused. "Err, you haven't been saying it the way it's said on my planet."

"I've been saying it wrong for seven years?"

"Loera, I don't say your name the way your parents do. Even I can hear the difference."

"But Hoban and Tthhooban sound nothing alike," she sputtered as she tried out the breathy sound.

Another shiver ran through Yaniqui. "Are there different types of dogs?" Her gaze avoided Loera.

Loera's eyes flashed. "Different types of dogs? My husband's been away for months rescuing you and you want a *dog*?"

"Loera…"

"Holoban," she stumbled on his name in front of the audience, "you've been gone. Gone to get her, and now she wants a dog. Great."

Oh shit. What a shitting shit storm. Hloban had to have seen this coming. And it wasn't fair to Yaniqui. Or Loera. And why couldn't Hloban see? Adam looked around. No one was going to step in.

"Yani," Adam said, "let me show you the stream." He pointed to the forest and tugged her along by the shirt she wore, borrowed a long time ago from Eeriva and never given back.

As they retreated, he heard, "Loera, it's going to be okay. She's shaken. I'm sorry I've been gone so long. We're going to—"

The uneven surface of the ground felt odd beneath their feet after the smooth manufactured ship floor. Adam stumbled over a stone and they walked in silence. He couldn't look at Yaniqui's face. He was pretty sure she was crying.

"It's through here," Adam said neutrally, as if everything was fine, and gestured toward the tree line. "This is Waquas's land. Well, the land the government leases to him. He's not allowed to own it, though he takes better care of it than they would."

Yaniqui trailed her fingers across the rough bark of a tree. This path was walked often. It was bared to the elements, and for that, slightly sticky with drying mud. A bird call rang through the forest.

At the end of the path, Adam jumped down a two-foot lip onto a sandy bank. He peeled his shoes and socks off. His feet looked desperate for sunlight. He walked a few steps forward and let the water rush gently over his skin.

"Yow!"

Yaniqui jumped back.

"What? What is it?"

"It's cold. Yowza. That's ice-cold."

A hysterical laugh escaped Yaniqui. "What is 'yowza' and how cold?"

"Just an expression. Try it out for yourself."

It was already chilly, but it was a relief to experience something other than the ship's constant temperature management. Yaniqui slipped off her shoes and set them neatly on the bank. She jumped down next to Adam and tentatively dipped one foot in.

"Ch-ch-ch," she stuttered. "That's freezing."

"You'll get used to it in a minute." Adam waded in a few more inches. "What do you think? About Earth, I mean."

"It's beautiful. The air is so clear. And this water. This amount of real water, nonmanufactured, it's a fortune."

"And we're just washing our smelly feet in it."

Yaniqui smiled. "There's more though, right? I don't mean the oceans, more small stuff like this?"

"It's everywhere. Most of us Earthlings don't give it a second thought. We learn in school that other planets don't have the same water resources as us, but that seems impossible."

"You Earthlings? Do you consider yourself one?"

"Of course. Until we went to get you, I had never been off-planet before. I'd never even been to our moon. This is my home."

The coldness was no longer so abrasive.

"But your dad is Wea Saavian."

"And my mom is an Earthling. Now this is his home planet too. Among Earthlings, there is a relatively wide variety of gene mutations because of the high diversity in ecosystems. People here have different-colored skin, different-colored hair, different facial features. I don't stand out as being other. Not at first anyway."

"It can be your home too. I'm serious."

Yaniqui grimaced.

Adam continued, "Listen, no one is under any delusions why you're here."

Yaniqui glared, but Adam pushed ahead. Someone had to.

"You came because you have nowhere else to go and hope to steal Hloban from Loera and fulfill your destiny. I'm not trying to be mean, but Loera will never let you win. Besides, they have a kid. You'll love Obani. Believe it or not, Loera is a nice person too. You need to move on."

The corners of Yaniqui's mouth tugged downward and she splashed the water with her foot. Tears welled in her eyes. Suddenly Adam was exhausted. After months in space, the gravity on Earth pulled at every part of him.

"I told him I'd let him go." More tears dripped and her voice dropped. "We were supposed to be together, but he never came for me. He got married and has this perfect life and mine was destroyed. How is that fair?"

"I don't know," Adam said quietly, "but I'm sorry for it."

# Chapter 36
## Yaniqui
## Earth

Yaniqui exhaled. This was not a bad place. Was this really it? Was this place going to keep her safe? When she had come face-to-face with Loera, she wished she had made Hloban and the others dump her at the first way station they came across. But this clean air... Yaniqui remembered the stifling air on the ship with her mother, after she had learned of her planet's demise. The dead air on the labor planet, as if you were part of a biological thing that had stopped working and since you were part of it, you were no longer working either. The violent air on Akar Evion. This clean air almost made all of it worth it.

She shivered.

"We should go back," Adam said. "I'm sure things are, uh, calmer now."

Yaniqui shrugged and picked up her shoes. She and Adam walked back barefoot.

"It's crazy," she said slowly. "I have no idea what tomorrow's going to look like. You'd think I'd be used to that by now."

Adam smiled. "I'm pretty sure tomorrow I'll wake up at my

parents' house. Go see my friends. But beyond that, I don't know what I'll be doing next week."

"It's weird, isn't it?"

"Yeah. But it's the best kind of beginning."

They were back in sight of the group. Amanda, Loera, and Keyad were talking in a tight-knit circle—Yaniqui could guess about what—and Hloban shadowed Obani as Waquas led them out of a field.

Yaniqui's impression of Loera was already that she was beautiful, but given the chance to covertly study her, it was clear she was elegant and confident as well. The bottom of Loera's twist out touched the tops of her shoulders. Her slouchy hunter green pants were casual but stylishly paired with a structured jacket, tiny flats, and artsy earrings.

She was more real than Yaniqui ever feared.

The air shifted as Yaniqui and Adam rejoined the group.

"It was very nice to meet you, Yaniqui." Amanda grinned and Yaniqui saw Adam reflected in her smile. "We'll have you over for dinner soon."

"It's going to be a huge adjustment," Keyad said, "but you'll get there. Anything you need—"

"You'll jump on a spacecraft and hop a few dozen star systems over to help me, I know." Yaniqui was joking, but she smiled shyly and gave Keyad an embrace. She thought she was going to cry again when they broke apart.

Adam was a little less easy. They agreed to get together soon so Adam could show her around town and introduce her to some friends. Whereas it would have been perfectly natural to part with a hug after weeks together, their avoidance hung in the air, a little sticky.

Yaniqui approached Waquas—he took her hand formally and wished her welcome one more time to Earth—and there was nothing left to do but get in the car with Hloban and his family. She rode in the back next to Obani, like a child. Loera acted as if she wasn't there and kept a running dialogue of things Hloban should know now that he was back—the nanny didn't work out so they'd gotten a new one named Carla who's fab, Obani played with his trains every day Hloban was gone, and Loera's parents want to take them out for dinner now that Hloban was home.

Obani studied Yaniqui's face bluntly as he made his assessments and interrupted his mother every once in a while to tell his dad some remembered story he'd been saving up for him.

Thoughts raced through Yaniqui's mind. Should she have insisted she be put up in a hostel until she found a permanent place to stay? They clearly had money. Was it too late to insist? But what if she couldn't figure out how to purchase food on this planet? What if they got separated again? What if Akar came for her?

Yaniqui looked out the window, jittery. All the hard things had to be behind her. She had to believe it.

Even in her trepidation, Yaniqui couldn't help peering at the houses, wondering about the lives of the people inside them. If this was any hint as to how Earthlings lived, they were incredibly lucky.

Finally, Loera pulled up to a gigantic white home. Yaniqui's mouth dropped open. They didn't have money, they were *rich*. Tiny yellow flowers dotted the walk to the front door. Loera pressed a button and a door revealed another vehicle inside the garage.

Obani seemed to have finally decided she was fine. "This is my house," he said.

They clambered out of the car and collected the few bags. Hloban was determined to take it all in one trip. Yaniqui brushed her sandy feet off, now dry. Loera opened the door and went inside without a look back and suddenly Yaniqui was in an eating area. She peered around at the cupboards and counters in near awe. Akar had luxury, but it was still space. There wasn't the room to spread out. This was extraordinary.

"Come see your room next," Obani shouted and bounded up the stairs. "I picked it all out!"

Yaniqui looked at Hloban to figure out what she should do. He looked at Loera who shrugged slightly.

"Sure, let's get you settled." She swallowed. "But don't worry, your room isn't filled with stuffed animals or neon curtains."

They all went up. Obani appeared briefly in one doorway, then ducked back in. Yaniqui pushed the rest of the door open. The walls were the palest of indigo. A pair of huge white closet doors flanked a couch for two and a tiny delicate end table. Yaniqui was gawking so much that she almost missed the bed. It stood square in an alcove. The bedding too was white, but a pale purple blanket lay elegantly at the foot of the bed.

"I picked this for you."

Obani held out a small ceramic dish with a little Earth creature in the middle, also ceramic. Yaniqui cradled it in her hand.

"It goes on a little table. For jewelry and coins and stuff. Just a little catchall." Loera wasn't quite looking at Yaniqui as she explained.

"This is—"

"Well, we'll let you get settled." Loera left and Obani darted after his mother.

Hloban walked up to Yaniqui, carefully, as if she were a Wipeout Con that could go off and destroy the pristine room. When she didn't look up, he grasped her lightly by the arms. "Welcome, Yaniqui. This is your home as long as you want it to be."

Yaniqui put another pancake on her plate. She let the tree sap—plant blood, a part of her whispered—spread across the plate. From what Yaniqui could tell, food in the galaxy was basically the same—the meat of other creatures and the fibers of those without consciousness. She amended that to include those that took light as their food source. And water was essential to many. So, four categories. She strained to think. *Was there a species that ate gases?* she wondered.

Loera sat at the other end of the table, drinking coffee and motioning quickly over a holo with a privacy setting that allowed Loera to see the text, images, or video that appeared, but all Yaniqui saw was a shimmering blue-gray square. Obani munched his pancakes happily. His father, Yaniqui mentally stumbled over the word, was still getting ready for the day.

Obani shocked Yaniqui more than Loera did. You could fight another woman. You couldn't change someone's parentage. That cemented it more than anything. Hloban was lost to her. Despite her angry feelings toward Obani's existence in the universe, she liked him. She couldn't help but laugh when he told Hloban that he was going to come and get him in space because he was taking so long.

But all the house felt too much like theirs. Photographs of Loera and Hloban hiking and drinking with friends. Hloban's handwriting on labels. Obani's baby footprints framed on the wall. And within it all, a room decorated specifically for the sweet young woman Loera had imagined.

When she crawled into bed the night before, Yaniqui was overwhelmed with relief that at last she had stopped moving. She didn't know if it was home yet, but she didn't have to run anymore. She thought longingly of Maemi and the pallet they had shared. Her mother who she may never see again. Who could be dead. Dissected and violated. It hurt so much. And yet, another made space to take care of *her*.

"Loera?"

Hloban's wife looked up warily. Her fingers moved a second longer and then she paused, waiting.

"You have a beautiful home. I'm very grateful for your family's help."

It took Loera a second to register Yaniqui's positive comment. A flicker of emotion crossed her face.

"I'm sorry I'm not what everyone was expecting," Yaniqui's eyes spilled over in a rush, and she covered her face, embarrassed. She put her fork down and started sobbing. Obani turned toward her with wide eyes but no embarrassment at watching a grown-up cry.

Loera was there then, and put an arm around Yaniqui. "Shh, it's okay. You're safe. You're here now and you're safe. We're going to help you."

Yaniqui nodded heavily and wiped her face.

"Besides," Loera said, looking Yaniqui right in the eye, "I make it a point to never be what anyone expects."

That afternoon, someone knocked lightly on Yaniqui's door. She sat in the window seat, writing in a large leather notebook. Yaniqui was surprised but pleased when Waquas had come to Hloban's house earlier that day and had given it to her. For the first time, she saw how objectively handsome he was and she wondered what life would be like if she let herself notice people other than Hloban.

"Yani?" Hloban asked.

She said without turning, "These are some shit sunsets."

Hloban laughed, caught off guard. "Well, they get pretty after a while. I know they're not the same. Is that what you were writing about?"

"Yeah," Yaniqui sighed.

"Really?"

"Well, partly. I'm writing everything I can remember about Wea Saa. Someone has to. Otherwise, it will exist only on the shelves of The Shou."

"You're right. We're the caretakers of what's left." Hloban flushed. "There might be a way to help prolong the memory of what we've lost though." Hloban didn't often stumble over his words. "I think that, oh, I'm just going to say it."

It was cute. Yaniqui smiled.

"I think you and Adam should get together."

The smile died on Yaniqui's face. She stood up, nestled the book on her bed, then turned to Hloban, fire in her eyes.

"Is *that* why you brought me here? To Earth? To be partners with the last single male from Wea Saa?" she spat. "You fucking *bastard*."

The fire flew out of Yaniqui as quickly as it had come when Hloban started crying. He sank to the edge of the bed and placed his hands over his eyes. She hadn't ever seen Hloban cry and she was overcome with shame. But still, she was offended.

"Yani, that's not it at all. You think that I would ever do that to you?" He sniffed. "This wasn't how it was supposed to be. You and me."

Yaniqui stayed silent.

"I spend every day with someone I love. But someone who's not my partner." Hloban spoke quietly now. "There are no partnerships here. Earth marriage sounds the same, but it's not. This is not perfect." Hloban took a deep breath. "But that doesn't mean this needs to be bad."

"Hloban, what you're asking of me—"

"—let me finish. Please. It's not about preserving bloodlines or stealing you to force you into something. It's…I…I'm the last person who knew you from before. I had a responsibility toward you and your family and I still do. But I can't take care of you. I can't be the person I thought I was going to be for you. But maybe I can help you have something close. I can't stand the thought of you living the rest of your life here, losing all touch with what you had as a heritage, and never speaking of it. But Adam could be that for you. It stands to reason that you're more compatible with him than anyone else on this planet." Hloban had control over his tears now.

Yaniqui rubbed a hand across one cheek. "I don't know. I feel like I don't want anything at all."

"Think about it, please. If there's a soul mate out there, that's not me…I have to believe it would be him."

# Chapter 37

Savini entered his private residence. In the face of the wealth of the Akar empire, what he was given was simple. It was a small space. His water allocation was half of what was allowed to newly acquired beings. He couldn't order food to his room like they could. But he didn't need any of that. Whereas the people around him were limited—the beings to their rooms, the workers to their departments—he could go anywhere, do anything.

When things were going well.

When they weren't going well, it was usually one person's fault.

That Wea Saavian.

He opened a cabinet, the only valuable thing in the room. Everything else was standard issue. He had brought the standing cabinet. Real sand pine wood with a dark inlay of shimmering olephen bone. The case was much more expensive than what it held inside.

Savini removed a heavy crystal glass and decanter of pale pink liquid, a shade lighter and brighter than the sand pine. He poured himself a measure, nothing more, and replaced the decanter. It was a rare drink, but only because there was no market for it. Nobody else wanted it.

The scent was heavy for a drink so lightly colored. It unfurled thickly through the room like waves of amber. He took a deep breath and sat down, a man in an expensive suit, holding an expensive glass on the same type of bed his inferiors slept on. The suit was a necessity. Akar wanted him to look powerful, set above the rest, but he knew in his bones he was as replaceable as the next promising captive.

At long last, he took a careful sip. It brought back flashes of the forest he lived in as a child. His mother pounding mavoc with a long-handled pestle, the pale pink root bruising but not breaking before it was submersed in nectar-flavored water.

It was a lifetime ago, and yet the few years he had spent in his mother's care felt more endless than the decades he had worked for Akar.

The room chirped. He set the still-full glass in his cabinet. He never rushed his drink. It would be there when he came back.

Outside his room, he walked down the long hall and opened a door to reveal the main command center. He was always just steps away from helping Akar fulfill its wishes.

He nodded at a tech who looked up from her work and stepped inside the side room. The clear glass automatically frosted over and all sounds outside the room deadened. A wave of light scanned the room for any unauthorized listening devices or equipment. It was the most private place on the spacecraft.

The screen buzzed to life.

Matts gave a toothy smile. They were always too pleased with themselves. "I'm in their star system now," they said without preamble.

"You're in *a* star system now. There's no proof that's where the Wea Saavian woman went. I don't want good news until you have it."

"Yes, sir."

"What's your timeline?"

"Travel is slow out here—but once I'm there, I expect things to escalate quickly."

Savini swallowed and fought the urge to put his head in his hands.

If Yaniqui could be his downfall, Matts could be his savior. It was a grim thought.

# Acknowledgements

I wrote the first scenes of *Dangerous to Heal* in 2013 in rural eSwatini as a Peace Corps Volunteer, scenes that I quickly outgrew thanks to the support and encouragement of many in my life.

Thank you to the team of beta readers that provided feedback on an early version of this book, including: Max DeMay, Alex Hellweg, Michael Kieffer, E. J. Solie, and Sarah Tyley. If a book is a window into another's soul, these fine friends and creators saw the gnarled, unedited foundations of mine.

Write On, Door County awarded me a writing retreat where I edited this book from dawn to bedtime for eight days. I appreciate their faith in me as a storyteller and all they do for the writing community.

I found great support in the industry professionals that helped me morph my story idea into a true book. Thank you to editors Dina Hemmons and Anne-Marie Rutella, and cover designer Andrew Davis.

I appreciate reader Brian Deyo for sharing his name with me and congratulate him one final time on winning my named character competition.

This book would be a shadow of itself without the endless wisdom of my book coach, Nicole Van Den Eng. She asked challenging questions that pushed my craft further and consulted on innumerable details of this book.

Finally, I am grateful for my husband, Oliver Zornow. Oliver has championed the art and ideas within this story for a decade and his powerful enthusiasm made all the difference.

# About the Author

Rebecca M. Zornow is the author of *It's Over or It's Eden* and *Dangerous to Heal*. She is a Hal Prize winner, a Peace Corps storytelling finalist, and has written for numerous print and digital publications.

Rebecca is an alumna of Lawrence University. After graduation, she served in the Peace Corps where she started school libraries and an art club in rural eSwatini. Rebecca is also a board member of the Caneille Regional Development Fund. She is a former magazine editor-in-chief and runs the book coaching business Conquer Books with writer and book coach Nicole Van Den Eng.

Learn more about Rebecca and sign up for her monthly newsletter at www.RebeccaMZornow.com.